The Caffeine Book

THE
CAFFEINE
BOOK

Frances Sheridan Goulart

DODD, MEAD & COMPANY   NEW YORK

Published by Dodd, Mead & Company, Inc.
79 Madison Avenue, New York, N.Y. 10016
Distributed in Canada by
McClelland and Stewart Limited, Toronto
Manufactured in the United States of America
First Edition

Library of Congress Cataloging in Publication Data

Goulart, Frances Sheridan.
  The caffeine book.

  Includes index.
    1. Caffeine habit.   2. Caffeine—Toxicology.
I. Title.
RC567.5.G68   1984   616.86′4   84-1602
ISBN 0-396-08371-4 (pbk.)

To my always-supportive family, Ron, Sean, and Steffan
And to Esme Carroll, who was always there

Contents

Introduction

Did you know that the world's most used and abused drug is one you take every day to start the day?

You may even take it in several forms *dozens* of times a day. Millions of Americans do.

The drug is caffeine, and the reason I've chosen to write about it is that it *is* so everyday, so acceptable, and so dangerous. Even the medical profession overlooks the role caffeine abuse plays in dozens of diseases, from chronic fatigue, the number one physical complaint in America today, to heart disease, the number one killer disease.

The second reason I've taken up the subject in detail is that, unlike killer diseases and addictions, such as alcoholism, the cure for caffeinism is simple and clear-cut. Kick the habit.

It is something most people can accomplish in six weeks. The payoff is improved mental and physical health. The price, if you don't or won't kick the habit, can be serious illness, even death.

The Caffeine Book

Chapter 1

Caffeine—The Great American Addiction

Caffeine—it's the all-American high. On any given day, Americans drink 450 million cups of coffee, and without fear of arrest or addiction.[1]

Coffee and the addictive drug it contains—caffeine—are legal. We use them and abuse them around the clock.

Coffee is a $4.8 billion business. In 1966 95% of us between the ages of 30 and 59 drank it. By 1981, consumption had slipped to 50%, but an estimated 90 million Americans are still regulars and 15 million of us are addicted to it to the tune of six or seven cups a day.[2, 3]

But caffeine comes in many other forms. And if you're average, you also get caffeine from cola and pepper-type soft drinks, tea, cocoa, chocolate, over-the-counter pep pills such as Vivarin, and many brands of aspirin, headache remedies, and even weight-loss aids, diuretics, and antihistamines.

Soft-drink consumption has skyrocketed in the last two decades, surpassing even coffee as America's favorite beverage, accounting for almost a tenth of the total calories in most diets.[4]

And much of the caffeine we consume comes from unsuspected sources. Noncola sodas, like Mello Yello and Mountain Dew, for example, contain as much caffeine as a cup of instant coffee.

We are a nation of coffeepot-heads, and 95% of all American families have the habit. For better or for worse, we drink more than 450 cups apiece each year. Most of us "get up" by being down in our cups seven days a week, even doctors. Only 17% of the medical profession surveyed abstains, says the Pan American Coffee Bureau, and almost seven out of ten Americans over ten years of age had at least one cup on a typical winter day in 1971.[5]

As a nation, we drink more coffee than any other country in the world—more than 50% of all the coffee that's produced. In per capita terms, however, we rank only eighth, behind the Swiss, Danes, Norwegians, Swedes, Belgians, Dutch, and French.[6] And yet certain segments of our coffee'd-up country stand out.

As a national group, American office workers drank more than 9 billion cups of java* on the job in 1981 alone. And odd-hour occupation groups tend to drink the most coffee of all. They include waitresses, night workers, theater people, and long-distance night drivers.[7]

The number of medical problems linked to coffee consumption is long and disturbing. It includes gastrointestinal ailments, heart disease, cancer, psychiatric disorders, kidney disease, low blood sugar, hyperactivity, even peri-

---

* The term "mocha java" is not really a synonym for coffee, although it is used that way. True mocha beans of any grade are exceedingly scarce. Grown on hillsides in the hot, dry climate of Arabia, they are the descendants of the dervish Omar and the goatherd Kaldi, and originally bedeviled both. What's more, very little coffee is still grown in Java, whose plantations were destroyed by the Japanese during World War II.

odontal bone loss. Caffeine is involved in day-to-day psychological problems, such as poor school performance by children, and adult employment problems caused by caffeine-induced fatigue, restlessness, and anxiety. Researchers have concluded that caffeine consumption is a physically and mentally burdensome cultural norm—a socially encouraged, subliminal drug addiction.

Including children, the average American consumes an average of 200 milligrams of caffeine each day—twice as much as it takes to produce significant bodily effects. It is estimated that 30% of us take in 500 to 600 milligrams of caffeine per day, and 10%, more than 1,000 milligrams per day, which is twice what doctors consider a large "drug dose."[8]

For some of us, caffeine could be fatal, if abused. "This drug [caffeine] should not be taken," cautions the *The Essential Guide to Prescription Drugs*, "if you have had an allergic reaction to any dosage form of it previously, have severe heart disease, or an active stomach ulcer. And only under a physician's care if you experience severe disturbances of heart rhythm, have a history of peptic ulcer disease, are subject to hypoglycemia, or have epilepsy."[9]

By definition, caffeine is a member of a group of chemicals called methylxanthines. It is also an alkaloid that occurs naturally in various amounts in many plant species, primarily those that are native to the tropics and subtropics. The best-known caffeine sources are coffee beans (about 1.3% caffeine, since the caffeine content varies from bean to bean and from leaf to leaf), tea leaves (up to 5%), kola (cola) nuts* (2.5%), *maté* (the gaucho drink—1%), and *guarana,* a South American drink made from seeds with three times the caffeine of coffee beans.

* Cola-type soft drinks have caffeine from the kola nut in addition to caffeine, which is added by the manufacturer.

Although caffeine is the strongest stimulant in coffee, tea, and cocoa, these drinks contain other xanthine compounds—theophylline and theobromine. They are related to caffeine but are less potent.

Other teas, or cola substitutes, which contain small but measurable amounts of noncaffeine stimulants include *maté* (or *matte*), passion flower, *kavakava,* and *gotu kola.*[10] It is the presence of theophylline in tea, for example, that can produce many of the same side effects as caffeine. It is suspected as the cause of the constipation often experienced by heavy tea drinkers. (More on theophylline in Chapter 4.)

That's not all. Your morning thunder could be disrupting your mental activity, say scientists at Prince Henry's Hospital in Melbourne, Australia. Their experiments have determined the existence of the chemical in coffee, which also acts as an opiate antagonist. Since the brain has naturally occurring opiates, the blockage of these "could produce mental depression, nervousness and anxiety," they say.

Dr. Paul Marangos, a biologist at the National Institute of Health, who has studied the effects of caffeine on brain physiology, concludes that caffeine blocks the brain's natural tranquilizers. Physiologically, notes Dr. Marangos, the brain responds to this blockage by producing an increase in the number of tranquilizer receptor sites. So when the effect of the caffeine wears off, coffee drinkers feel even more tired than they would otherwise feel.[11]

A further undesirable disease-producing chemical is tannin, found in varying amounts in tea and coffee (see page 64 for details). Coffee also contains other toxic substances unrelated to caffeine (see Chapter 2).

Caffeine, says the *Newsletter of the Institute for Nutri-*

tional Research, is an alkaloid, and alkaloids are the active principles of many plants, often medicinal ones. Among them, besides caffeine, are such compounds as strychnine, atropine, hyoscine, theobromine, and nicotine. Some, such as nicotine, are so poisonous that, if not largely destroyed by the burning of the cigarette, would certainly kill the smoker. All members of this family cause a state of physical dependency or addiction in users.[12]

Caffeine* is the mildest of the habit-forming drugs—but it is still medically classified with other drugs, such as opiates, amphetamines, alcohol, and barbiturates.

Caffeine's drug action begins in approximately 30 minutes, and reaches a maximum in 50 to 75 minutes. So do some of the side effects, notes James W. Long in *The Essential Guide to Prescription Drugs.* Caffeine's side effects are "natural, expected and unavoidable drug actions" and include nervousness, insomnia, increased urine output, headache, irritability, lightheadedness, feeling of drunkenness, impaired thinking, nausea, heartburn, indigestion, stomach irritation, and development of stomach ulcer. Tolerance for caffeine often decreases after the age of 60, making the drinker more susceptible to the development of the side effects cited.

"Thus we come to the coffee paradox—the question of how a drug so fraught with *potential* hazard can be consumed in the United States at the rate of more than a hundred billion doses a year . . . without doing intolerable damage—and without arousing the kind of hostility, legal repression, and social condemnation aroused by the illicit drugs" asks one group. "The answer is quite simple. Coffee,

---

* It has been speculated that the flavor and aroma of the brewed coffee bean—independent of the caffeine—has helped make coffee such an object of desire, observed one researcher.

tea, cocoa, and the cola drinks have been *domesticated*. Caffeine has been incorporated into our way of life in a manner that minimizes (though it does not altogether eliminate) the hazards inherent in caffeine use."[13]

Surveys indicate most of us think of caffeine as a nondrug. At least, that's what we tell ourselves and each other.

In a detailed study published in 1969 by Dr. Avram Goldstein and Dr. Sophia Kaizer of the Department of Pharmacology, Stanford University School of Medicine, 239 young married women were asked why they drank coffee in the morning. The vast majority (72%) gave the usual answers suggesting that coffee is a nondrug, the researchers reported. They "enjoyed it" or they "liked the taste."[14]

Yet, nearly a third of the participants also admitted they were dependent on coffee. Here are five reasons given by 25 housewives who drank coffee *before* breakfast: "helps you wake up," "gets you going in the morning," "gives you a lift," "stimulates you," and "gives you energy."

What Caffeine Does

What happens when you drink a cup of coffee? Here is what is behind that biochemical buzz you go for every day.

1. The caffeine you get in coffee, tea, or cola is absorbed immediately, and its effects are felt within half an hour. Peak blood levels are reached about 60 minutes after consumption, then fade in about 3½ hours. (Peak levels may be reached in less than 3½ hours or later, depending on the individual's age, sex, and health. Likewise, the effects begin to fade anywhere from 1 to 2½ hours after peaking.)

2. Caffeine works by stimulating the brain—both the

6

central cortex, which handles thought processes, and the medulla, which regulates heart rate, respiration, and muscular coordination. This nervous assault produces "coffee nerves" and that jumpy, "hyper" feeling associated with overconsumption. Caffeine also raises the body's metabolic rate slightly, increasing the number of calories the body burns. But it also triggers the release of insulin, causing blood sugar to fall, producing feelings of hunger and letdown.

3. Caffeine stimulates the heart muscle. At high doses, it can cause a hazardously rapid beat. Coronary arteries dilate, increasing blood flow to the heart, and blood vessels feeding the brain constrict, reducing cerebral blood flow.

4. Caffeine also relaxes the muscles in the respiratory system, the digestive tract, and the kidneys, causing increased urination. Because caffeine is a diuretic, it has a dehydrating effect on the body. Large amounts of coffee can cause diarrhea, while tea leads to constipation. Caffeine affects the heart in much the same manner as it abuses the nerve centers. The heart beats more forcefully. This is the stimulating (irritating) effect. But when the drug is finally expelled from the body, the heart beats with less force. When the blood pressure is increased, additional strain is placed on the kidneys. Coffee has a congesting effect. Kidney congestion results in an increase of urine output, and the kidneys try to expel the various coffee poisons. If coffee drinking is continued and/or increased, this congestion weakens the kidneys, and ultimately kidney function degenerates. This may lay the foundation for other chronic diseases, not necessarily of the kidneys, in later years.

5. While caffeine makes voluntary muscles less easily fatigued, it improves the capacity for muscular work and

increases the speed and efficiency of mental and manual tasks, while improving concentration. A clearer train of thought may result, a keener appreciation of sensory stimuli, and a swifter reaction time. Studies indicate that after two cups of coffee, driving skills improve, and manual tasks, such as typing, speed up.

Caffeine affects the walls of the blood vessels in the wake-sleep center and thought-association areas of the brain. By increasing the energy level of the chemical systems responsible for nerve-tissue activity, it induces wakefulness and improves alertness and mental acuity.[15] But is it worth the risk?

Studies show that a single drop of concentrated caffeine will produce death in minutes when injected into the skin of a small animal; a tiny amount injected into its brain will bring on convulsions.[16]

According to Dr. Solomon Snyder, director of neuroscience at the Johns Hopkins School of Medicine, the compound adenosine is a building block of DNA and a neuromodulator, or nerve depressant, that is blocked by caffeine and, to a lesser extent, by theobromine and theophylline.

In addition, like the "hard drugs," caffeine causes a nerve center known as locus ceruleus, located near the top of the spinal cord, to malfunction. The ceruleus is involved with control of heart rate and respiration. It also stimulates many parts of the brain. While heroin pacifies the user by slowing down this group of neurons, the caffeine and theophylline in coffee cause them to overreact, reports Dr. D. E. Redmond of Yale University's Neuro-Behavioral Laboratory. Halting the drug, in either case, leads to withdrawal symptoms experienced by the reformed users.[17]

The amount of caffeine in a single cup of coffee is admittedly small. But very few of us stop after one cup. Most of us have at least two and a half cups in the course of a day.[18] And one-fourth of the population drinks five or more cups of coffee a day.

This cumulative "caffeine overload" gradually overburdens various systems of the body, the nervous and eliminative systems in particular, especially if the system is already weakened by poor health, for example, the presence of diabetes, heart disease, or arthritis.

Caffeine has only recently been recognized as the psychoactive chemical it is. And not everybody agrees on its dangers. For example, some researchers believe caffeine has its contributions to make to our well-being, outside of its few legitimate medical uses.

According to David Costill of the Human Performance Laboratory in Madison, Wisconsin, a little coffee before athletic competition is beneficial. In his study of the effects of caffeine on athletic performance, he has found that a couple of cups of coffee on the morning of a race increases the ability to perform work by as much as 16%, depending on the individual. Caffeine—about the amount found in two cups of coffee, or 200 milligrams—seems to aid the body in burning fat, which will spare glycogen in the muscles.

Costill estimates that although caffeine is a drug, only about 20% of the population may have a negative reaction to caffeine, such as a bad case of the jitters.[19]

Coffee is a white-collar helper, too. Several years ago, researchers for the Federal Injury Control Research Laboratory in Rhode Island found that typists with a cup of coffee on their desks type faster and make fewer mistakes than those without coffee. The same study found the equivalent of two to four cups of coffee improved the driving abilities of 24 male drivers it tested.[20]

Caffeine has legitimate medical uses as well. It is valuable as a cardiovascular and pulmonary stimulant and as a diuretic. It can be used to relieve headaches following medical spinal punctures because it constricts the blood vessels in the brain and decreases the flow of cerebral blood.

Two other good uses for this drug are cited by *New York Times* health reporter Jane E. Brody: "Caffeine can be an alternative to potent and dangerous drugs used to treat hyperactive children. In some studies two cups of coffee daily had a paradoxical calming effect on such children, resulting in improved behavior and school performance. . . . Caffeine is also being used to treat premature babies who have attacks of apnea, or who periodically stop breathing in their sleep. Apnea, if not corrected in time, can result in sudden infant (crib) death. Caffeine may prevent these episodes of apnea and produces a more regular breathing pattern in such infants."[21]

Dr. Tom Ferguson, editor of *Medical Self Care,* cites another: "Caffeine helps to abort migraines in some people, although it can trigger headaches in others. And while caffeine is able to raise body temperature, it also interferes with aspirin's anti-fever action, say researchers. Avoiding tea, coffee, and colas as well as caffeine-containing medications when you have a fever may be wise."

Another good word for caffeine comes from the U.S. Department of Agriculture, which is studying coffee and cacao beans, because of their ability to resist contamination by mycotoxins and other poisons produced by fungi. The key, according to the department, is the caffeine that is abundant in both coffee and cacao beans. Most other tropical and semitropical foods, when improperly stored in

10

hot, humid climates, can develop molds, such as aflatoxins, which are carcinogenic. The Department of Agriculture is still trying to find out what causes caffeine to thwart the growth of the fungi.[22]

Caffeinism

Everything that goes up must come down.

Caffeine's primary effects are good: a temporary sense of well-being, a feeling of being "high," relief from fatigue, and stimulation of the nerves.

It is followed by so-called secondary effects, which aren't so good: from simple letdown to mental and physical depression, nervous exhaustion, decreased muscular power, and serious damage to the liver and kidneys.

And that dreaded secondary feeling of letdown is what leads to the second cup, and when it leads to several more cups, you're hooked. When caffeine—whatever its source—makes you feel so good you don't want to stop, the trouble starts. It explains why we consume 2 billion pounds of coffee a year.[23]

Is Caffeine Addictive?

If you're no good without your morning coffee or tea, you have plenty of drug-addicted company. For example, according to Dr. John Minton of Ohio State University, when forty-seven of his female patients were given a choice between totally eliminating caffeine from their diet or undergoing surgery for removal of breast lumps caused by caffeine intake, twenty-seven of them opted for surgery.

At one time the coffee-addiction syndrome used to be called "coffee nerves." Now it's more often called caffein-

11

ism, or chronic caffeine intoxication.* The symptoms of caffeinism, according to Dr. John F. Greden, a psychiatrist at the University of Michigan, read like a classic description of an anxiety attack: nervousness, anxiety, irritability, muscle twitching, jitteriness, and insomnia (see Chapter 8).

Six percent of all Americans suffer caffeinism severe enough to require professional treatment. And according to Dr. Kirby Gilliland and Dr. Gordon Deckert of the University of Oklahoma, authorities on the disorder, 15% of the country's coffee drinkers suffer from "undiagnosed caffeinism."[24]

Drinking more than ten cups of coffee per day (about 1,000 milligrams of caffeine) can produce frightening sensory disturbances, such as ringing in the ears, spots before the eyes, or even hallucinations, says Sanford Bolton, Ph.D., of St. John's University in New York City. Even if you have never experienced any of these symptoms, you're still not in the clear. You've probably just built up a tolerance to coffee. Year after year of heavy caffeine ingestion always takes its toll somewhere.[25]

The presumed danger point, above which one is at high risk, is 200 to 750 milligrams. The dose that may do it, in other words, is equal to drinking about three cups of coffee per day, or six cups of tea or cocoa, or eleven small glasses of cola drink.[26] According to a study by scientists at Vanderbilt University with six men and three women aged 21 to 30, all noncoffee drinkers, caffeine in this amount increased the average adrenaline output by 207%, and the norepinephrine output, by 75%. The blood pressure increased by a tenth, the respiratory rate shot up by

* One of the first descriptions of caffeinism appeared in the December 1967 issue of the *Journal of the American Medical Association*.

20%, and the heart rate dropped slightly at first, then increased after about an hour.[27]

Another side effect of caffeinism is what's called cross-addiction. According to a study conducted by the University of Michigan Medical School among depressed psychiatric patients, half of the seven-cup-or-more a day drinkers were also heavy users of cigarettes and alcohol and showed a higher rate of addiction to marijuana, tranquilizers, and various hypnotic drugs.

The Caffeine Controversy

The news that caffeine is irresistible but unhealthy is hardly news. And there is nothing twentieth-century about coffee addiction either.

There is Bach's *Coffee Cantata,* in which the heroine pleads with her father, "If I can't have my little demitasse of coffee three times a day, I'm just like a dried-up piece of roast goat!"

In the 18th century, Brillat-Savarin, the renowned French gastronome who praised coffee often, once warned, "It is the duty of all papas and mamas to forbid their children coffee, unless they wish to have little dried-up machines stunted and old at the age of 20."

And Sir James MacKintosh, the Scottish philosopher and statesman, claimed that the powers of a man's mind were directly proportional to the quantity of coffee he drank. . . . not to mention Frederick the Great, the Prussian monarch who, according to legend, often had his coffee made with champagne instead of water.

But what *is* news is that as dangerous as caffeine has been shown to be, it has become an ingredient in many commonly used foods, drinks, and drugs. Lately, our intentions have been in the right place. Jane E. Brody points to "the declining consumption of regular coffee, the steep rise in the proportion of decaffeinated coffees, the explosive growth of herbal teas, and the recent introduction of ordinary teas stripped of caffeine."

The decline in the use of caffeine began in 1978, when an advisory committee to the U.S. Food and Drug Administration (FDA) reported that too much caffeine might have a deleterious effect on central nervous system development. Since then, several studies have linked caffeine with birth defects, fibrocystic breast disease (a benign disorder), and pancreatic cancer.

Consumer groups have called for a ban on products, or, at the very least, prominent labeling on products to which caffeine has been added. Understandably, the soft-drink and coffee industries, afraid of raising public fear and losing business, have fought back.

Between the pro-caffeine and anticaffeine forces there is the FDA, in charge of providing us with the truth. After four years of debate and testing, no absolute answers are available to satisfy everyone.

Has our perception of caffeine as a potential hazard had an impact on the coffee industry? It seems so.

According to the National Coffee Association (NCA), comprising the roasters and others allied with the industry, 75% of the population drank coffee in 1962; in 1982, the figure had dropped to 56%. Thirty years ago, coffee consumption was 3.1 cups per person per day; in 1981 it was 1.9 cups.[28]

And while we are drinking more caffeine-laced soft drinks, we are drinking more decaffeinated coffee, too. Sales of decaffeinated coffee are up 15% since 1962. Decaffeinated coffee and coffee mixtures account for 15% of all the coffee purchased, says the International Coffee Organization (ICO). Likewise, when Royal Crown introduced RC100, a decaffeinated, sugar-free beverage in 1980, sales tripled in 12 months. Estimates are that between 15 and 20 million cases were sold in 1981.

Following the lead of the leaders, Sunkist also began to phase caffeine out of its formula in 1981, although, as of the spring of 1981, caffeine-containing versions were still on many shelves.

Because 7-Up's campaign involved "We're caffeine free, the others aren't"—comparative advertising claims—the Pepsi company responded by threatening to cancel its exclusive franchises of bottlers who participated in 7-Up's ad campaign. At that point the Federal Trade Commission began investigations for possible antitrust violators. (See Chapter 5 for complete details on caffeinated soft drinks.)

Governing Caffeine

"If caffeine were a newly synthesized drug, the manufacturers would have great difficulty getting it licensed for sale ... and if it were licensed, it would certainly be available only by prescription," says Dr. Tom Ferguson.[29]

Caffeine is one of the few drugs—like alcohol and quinine—that shouldn't, but does, show up throughout our food supply. And caffeine is probably the *only* dangerous drug that is widely available everywhere to children of all ages—and in a variety of forms—without a prescription.

It is painfully clear why nobody does anything. Like many food laws, the law governing caffeine in our food supply does more to protect the interests of manufacturers than the interests of the consumers.

"If the evidence is very clear, I'd have to act," said Jere

15

E. Goyan, the new Commissioner of Food and Drugs in an interview in 1982. "But if we are not certain, then the economic and political factors are certainly important. If we were to move against caffeine, and then 6 to 12 months later the studies were refuted, we would lose credibility. It's a balance act all the way."[30]

How does the FDA feel about caffeine?

"We're not saying it's unsafe, we're just not saying it's safe," says Dr. Sanford Miller, director of the FDA's Bureau of Foods.

Will reading labels help you avoid caffeine or reduce intake? In the case of coffee, tea, chocolate, and cocoa—no. Caffeine and related stimulants occur naturally in these foods. If it has been removed or reduced, the manufacturer will say so on the label. In the case of drugs and soft drinks—yes. Both over-the-counter drugs and prescribed medications must note on the label or enclosures both the presence of caffeine and the amount. There is, however, no way of knowing from the label how much caffeine is present from one cola to the next, although the difference may be as great as 10 milligrams or more (see Tables 7, 8, and 10).

The U.S. Department of Agriculture allows no more than 3 milligrams per ounce of caffeine to be added to diet soda, or 6 milligrams per ounce to regular cola drinks.

Caffeine is also found in anything the government considers a "pepper" drink, so it is possible to get that cola "kick" from orange, apple, and other fruit-flavored sodas classified a "pepper" type pepper-upper.

What's being done to alter a law that sanctions an unsafe substance?

Until 1978, caffeine was on the government's GRAS (Generally Recognized As Safe) list, along with hundreds

16

of substances. Then the Federation of American Societies for Experimental Biology, an FDA scientific advisory group, studied the literature on caffeine as part of its review of the GRAS list of food additives. The group was concerned with the effect of caffeine on children, who, because of their body size, require less caffeine than adults for side effects to show up.

Chronic consumption by some children of caffeine from cola-type drinks might impair brain or central nervous system development, but the federation said it did not know precisely what consumption levels might be dangerous. It recommended that caffeine be removed from the GRAS list and placed in an interim category until tests on its safety could be concluded. As late as 1982, those charges were still pending.

"Most of the 415 food additives that have been used by processors for years have been found to be safe, but some . . . may require stricter controls," said the FDA on December 30, 1980. "Salt, one of the most widely used of all food ingredients, was classified with additives that the scientists said should be more tightly restricted or even prohibited from use. . . . And caffeine was also included in a category of substances for which additional studies were recommended."[31]

It is expected that caffeine will soon be an optional ingredient, even though the FDA insists the evidence linking caffeine and numerous health hazards is not conclusive.

On the other hand, decaffeinated products are already available in both supermarkets and health food stores.

What does this mean?

The new "interim" status proposed for caffeine may have little practical effect for several years. Removing caffeine from the GRAS list means that food manufacturers would no longer be allowed to develop *new* uses for caffeine at will, but that it could still be used in all types of foods where it is presently added—until research has resolved the major safety questions.

Chapter 2

What You Need to Know About Coffee

"Coffee makes a sad man cheerful; a languorous man, active; a cold man, warm; a warm man, glowing; a debilitated man, strong. It intoxicates, without inviting the police; it excites a flow of spirits, and awakens mental powers thought to be dead.... When coffee is bad, it is the wickedest thing in town; when good, the most glorious.... The very smell of coffee in a sick room terrorizes death," observed social historian John Ernest McCann in 1902.

And the French nineteenth-century statesman Talleyrand insisted on having his coffee "black as the devil; hot as hell; pure as an angel and sweet as love."

Today, at any given second, Americans drink 4,848 cups.[1] New Yorkers alone drink 2 million cups of coffee every 20 minutes.[2]

While only 37% of us smoke, 80% of us drink coffee. That includes 50% of all Americans over the age of 10, and 83% of the medical profession.[3] One-half of all the coffee produced in the world is consumed annually in the United States.[4]

And there are more than 200 ground-coffee products representing nearly 100 brands to choose from in the nation's supermarkets.[5]

Yet coffee is a study in contradiction. Ten billion pounds of it are produced annually, making coffee the most significant single commodity in the western hemisphere. Yet, every coffee bean is still picked by hand.[6] (A coffee berry contains two kernels, or "beans." These are separated from the outer layers of the berries, then dried, graded, and shipped green in burlap sacks to roasters' warehouses.)

It keeps the economy alive—coffee is America's largest agricultural import and the second largest import, after petroleum. And yet, seventy cups of it can kill a man, while seven cups can produce acute toxic effects.[7]

It's even a poison that prevents poisoning. According to recent studies by the Department of Agriculture, thanks to the caffeine in the bean, coffee is the only tropical plant that is able to resist contamination by mycotoxins, such as aflatoxins, which are carcinogenic.[8]

At the very least, it can lead you to drink—the other kind—even though, ironically, black coffee is supposed to be what keeps you sober. According to a study by Dr. Patricia Mutch of Michigan State University, two groups of rats had the same diet, with one group also getting the equivalent of nine cups of coffee a day. When both groups had a choice between sugared water or sweetened alcohol, the coffee-drinking animals always picked the alcohol.[9]

In fact, coffee is not a bean *or* a legume. It is the fruit of a semitropical evergreen. "Few people know that coffee is a fruit product," points out the National Coffee Association. "The coffee tree bears a flower of breathtaking beauty, looking much like an orange blossom and heavy with jasmine-like fragrance. Its fruit not only resembles our North American edible cherry, but it actually is called a cherry.

In the case of our cherry, we eat the pulpy part and discard the pit. It's the other way around in the coffee cherry, where the pulp is thrown away and the bean inside is used to make the brew.... The average tree bears about 2,000 cherries, enough to produce only a single pound of roasted coffee."[10]

Coffee Beans: Nutritional and Food Value

According to an old Dutch proverb, "Coffee has two virtues—it is wet and warm." That's still true. In fact, in the opinion of many researchers and nutritionists, that's still all coffee has to offer.

If coffee were a food, say nutritionists, it would contain something that the body could utilize in the repair, maintenance, and replacement of tissues, or in the performance of its various functions. That's how a food is defined. But coffee doesn't. Its long-term effect on the body is catabolic (which means it tears down). Although the chief culprit is caffeine, coffee has many other toxic substances: volatile oils that irritate the delicate lining of the intestinal tract, creosote, pyridine, and tar. All are harmful to the body, primarily affecting the stomach, liver, heart, nervous system, and kidneys.

Certain kinds of tar, for example, produce cancer, too. The tar from tobacco products produces cancer in laboratory animals. Tar is also found in coffee. And it has the same physical characteristics as tobacco. In one study, 73% of laboratory animals treated with this coffee tar developed malignant tumors. Definite sores in the stomachs and digestive tracts also occurred. The roasting of coffee produces these tars. They are not soluble in water, so perhaps they are not present in coffee as we drink it. Still, in chemical tests such as spectrography and luminescence analysis,

21

coffee tars show the same characteristics as coal tar. But no studies have established a link between tar and human tumors.

Nevertheless, coffee does qualify technically as a food. It was, in fact, once eaten as a protein and fermented for wine, according to food historian James Trager.[11] Its bitter, somewhat astringent flavor is the result of the more than 500 volatile compounds it contains. According to the Internal Flavors and Fragrances Bureau, the coffee bean is the most complex naturally occurring flavor in the world.

Coffee is a fair source of niacin and contains traces of the other B vitamins. It is moderately rich in some essential minerals. A cup of prepared Sanka has 120 milligrams of potassium, and a cup of regular instant coffee has 81 milligrams. (That beats the 46 milligrams in beer and the 1.3 milligrams in ginger ale.)

Instant coffee also contains 2,068 milligrams of magnesium per pound of powder, almost as much as wheat bran and more than many magnesium-rich nuts. But ironically, coffee leads to diarrhea, and for many, heavy drinking leads to magnesium deficiency.

Coffee also has less sodium than soft drinks, beer, apple cider, or milk. One cup of milk, for example, contains 127 milligrams of sodium, while a cup of instant coffee has less than 3 milligrams.

Coffee takes away far more nutrients than it contributes to the diet. According to the Center for Science in the Public Interest, located in Washington, D.C., which surveyed doctors, dieticians, and allergists before compiling its ratings, coffee is number four on the ten worst foods list because it is "a vitamin antagonist." The vitamins it destroys the most are the water-soluble B-complex and ascorbic acid (vitamin C).

On the other hand, if it does nothing much to nourish your body, it may help your snap beans grow. Coffee grounds are almost as rich as early-cut alfalfa in nitrogen phosphate and potassium; combined with a material high in carbon or fiber, it makes a first-rate garden compost.

But nutrients aside, coffee's food values are endangered by the fact that coffee isn't a clean bean. Large quantities of the beans are rejected every year by the FDA. "Decomposed coffee beans are mixed purposely with first-grade beans while insect-laden bags are slipped through when investigators are off guard," say FDA officials.[12]

Green coffee detained by import inspectors increased from about 20 million pounds in 1972 to 83.5 million pounds in 1975. Live and dead insects among the beans accounted for 52% of the inspections-detentions in 1976, and bird and rodent excreta were responsible for 12%. "Debris such as bits of metal are still persistently present in many shipments," say government reports.[13]

Worse, according to investigations by Senator Gaylord Nelson (Democrat of Wisconsin), the FDA has found traces of six pesticides in coffee imported from twelve countries, four of which have been banned in the United States because they cause cancer in laboratory animals.

How does this happen? "An oft-forgotten loophole in the Federal Insecticide, Fungicide and Rodenticide Act makes it possible for American companies to produce pesticides for export, even after their use has been banned in the United States," says the Center for Science in the Public Interest. "So dozens of pesticides are sent abroad to countries where regulations are weak and rarely enforced. Among those countries receiving the pesticides are the ten biggest suppliers of coffee to the United States."

Adds the *FDA Consumer*, "Less common, but more hazardous, is chemical contamination. Lots of coffee from Colombia has been detained because the beans were shipped contaminated with several different chemicals, including ferrosilicon concentrate and lead sulfide. [One shipment of] coffee, valued at over $2.5 million, was detained during entry at the Port of San Francisco."[14]

The caffeine in coffee is good for getting you going, but when you learn what else it is good for, you may wish you hadn't gone. According to Lewis E. Machatka, writing in the *Better Life Journal*, "Coffee contains tannic acid, the stuff used for tanning leather from animal hides. Coffee is an excellent cleanser for greasy and dirty kitchen floors, stainless steel tables, deep fryers, butcher blocks ... any grease-covered surface. Coffee even cleans white-wall tires better than the chemicals recommended for that use."[15]

Industrial applications other than cleansing? "The Afghanistanis make coffee, put it in pans around their buildings, and since water is so short the rats drink it and die."

Even if the beans are good when they reach the docks, they may be bad by the time *you* get them. "Coffee beans contain 10 to 15 percent oil," says Manhattan's Coffee Bureau Brewing Center, "and stale residues become rancid and taint a new batch in a few days."[16]

Coffee in History

"Coffee would not be approved today if it were being presented to the Federal Food and Drug Administration for consideration. Once tests of it were completed and all of the side effects honestly evaluated, it would probably be confined to a doctor's prescription only," writes Ray Josephs in *Nutrition Health Review*.[17]

Indeed, although coffee is as "street legal" as pasteurized milk, and drunk more often, it has not always been so.

The use of the coffee bean as food, drink, and stimulant goes back approximately 1,000 years. The raw fruit of the coffee plant was used to make the first caffeinated beverage, which, legend has it, was a wine. And since raw coffee beans are considerably stronger than roasted ones, coffee was probably even more health-hazardous and highly addictive then than any caffeinated concoction today.

Not until two or three years later did someone suggest roasting the coffee bean to mellow the flavor and improve the aroma.

Coffee didn't evolve into the hot drink we know until A.D. 1000. And we have the Arabs (some say Omar Khayyam was the first java junkie) to thank for our addiction.

The Turks, who held a monopoly on coffee cultivation until the seventeenth century, sold the devil's brew to the Venetians, who opened coffeehouses in Venice on the Piazza San Marco as early as the end of the century. From Venice, the drink spread to France. "In a society whose medicine was based on herbs, hope and prayer, coffee—whose caffeine brightened the eye and revved up the mind—was a natural," observes researcher Carol Ann Rinzler.[18]

The French said coffee cured smallpox, gout, and scurvy. The English claimed it prevented death and cured indigestion, venereal disease, even the common cold. And English ladies, who were barred from English coffeehouses, said it made men impotent.

Some Muslim sects advocated coffee to improve religious diligence, while other faiths considered coffee drink-

25

ing to be a devotional lapse. By the end of the 1600s, coffee drinking gained ground in Europe and then made its way to North America.

Coffeehouses first appeared in Colonial America about 1670. The word *café*, which means coffee in French, Spanish, and Portuguese, derives from the old coffeehouse. Another word derived from coffee is "cafeteria," a combination of *café*, meaning coffee, and *teria*, meaning shop.

But our cups haven't always runneth over with coffee here. Tea, in fact, introduced to the Western world by China, was the major stimulating beverage until the famous Boston Tea Party.

Not only did American colonists dump tea into Boston's bay, but they also switched to drinking coffee.

Caffeine has been a source of public concern longer than most of the public realizes. In 1825, the gastronome Brillat-Savarin observed, "Coffee is a far more powerful liquor than is commonly believed. A man of sound constitution may drink two bottles of wine a day, and live long; the same man would not so long sustain a like quantity of coffee; he would become imbecile or die of consumption."[19]

Coffee hasn't always been as legal as water either. Some of the more orthodox Muslims believed that it was an intoxicating beverage and hence prohibited by the Koran: severe penalties were threatened to those addicted to its use.

Dr. Robert S. de Ropp notes that when coffee was introduced into Egypt in the sixteenth century, "The 'coffee bugaboo' . . . caused almost as much fuss as the 'marijuana bugaboo' in [the] contemporary United States. Sale of coffee was prohibited; wherever stocks of coffee were found they were burned."[20]

Coffee has been attacked by twentieth-century observers as well. In his book *Morphinism and Narcomanias From Other Drugs,* Dr. T. D. Crothers, superintendent of the Walnut Lodge Hospital in Connecticut, editor of the *Journal of Inebriety,* and professor of nervous and mental diseases at the New York School of Clinical Medicine, put coffee addiction in a class with morphinism and alcoholism.

Crothers charged that coffee could cause psychosis, adding that "in some extreme cases, delusional states of a grandiose character appear.... Associated with these are suspicions of wrong and injustice from others."[21]

What gave coffee its big boost in the United States was national Prohibition, imposed by the Volstead Act of 1919.

As Frederick Lewis Allen noted in *Only Yesterday,* at that time you could still buy a cup of coffee for a nickel, and the ban on the sale of alcoholic beverages, which lasted until 1933, led millions to the brink of a coffee cup. Temperance organizations campaigned against coffee as well as alcohol throughout the 1920s.

Until World War I, Europe was coffee's biggest customer. But by 1934, the United States was importing 50% of the world supply, and by 1940, with Europe at war, U.S. imports accounted for better than 70% of the world crop.

Instant Coffee

According to the International Coffee Organization, a London-based group representing the world's seventy coffee-producing and coffee-consuming nations, 32.5% of all the coffee sold today is in instant form.[22] Compared to most other caffeinated forms of drink, it is a relative newcomer. The processing is what makes it so different from regular brew.

Patents for liquid extracts and essences of coffee, and

even powders, go back to the last century. But the first commercially successful powdered coffee was not produced until 1906, when G. Washington's Red E Coffee, a "soluble" coffee, was produced in a plant in Brooklyn, New York.

Today, 90% of the instant coffee sold in America is sold by General Foods, Procter & Gamble, and Nestlé.

Here's how it's made. Huge amounts of coffee—up to 2,000 pounds at a time (up to 55% of the bean) are percolated in the factory. The soluble parts are extracted, and this coffee "juice" then is shot through tubes where high pressure and intense heat produce a coffee-extract concentrate. Step two is dehydration.

For powdered instant, the extract is dried in air heated to 500° F. This evaporates the water, leaving a finely grained instant coffee, which is remoistened slightly to create clumps that will dissolve readily in hot water. It is then packed into jars.

For freeze-dried coffees, the extract is frozen, broken into granules, and placed in a vacuum dryer, and the frozen water is transformed directly into vapor, which is removed. The remaining coffee granules dissolve instantly in hot water.

The processing pretty much explains why instant coffee doesn't taste like regular. Instant coffee gets cooked too much, and the redolence of the roasted bean creates a caramel flavor. Few of the volatile oils that account for aroma and taste are left. "A variety of ingenious techniques are used to recover the lost aromatic compounds. . . ." says Consumers Union. "Aromatization gives instant coffee more coffee aroma, but, because of oxidation, the aroma is bound to fade long before the coffee in the jar is used up."

What's worse, the Consumers Union continues, "American manufacturers often buy the cheapest (and usually the worst) coffee beans to keep the price of their product low. Why spend extra money on beans, especially for instant coffee, when the beans are going to be so heavily processed? The undesirable taste and aroma . . . can be attributed at least in part to the use of cheap beans."[23]

Freeze-dried coffees retain more of the coffee bean's flavor because they are subjected to less heat than regular instant coffee.

One reason decaffeinated coffee is lower in caffeine is that so much of the bean can be dissolved when roasted and ground coffee is brewed. The extra quantity of dissolved bean is largely soluble fiber and aroma-free, with only a trace of caffeine. More total product with minimal caffeine results in a smaller overall percentage of caffeine in the final product.

Special Coffees

"Espress yourself! It's simple. Your dinners have a special afterglow when you espress your compliments to your guests. . . . You can make Medaglia d'Oro. . . ." says the ad.

It may be simple, but espresso and dark-roasted after-dinner type brews, such as Macchinetta, are not the better ways of going after an afterglow.

Espresso is a very dark roasted coffee that is preferred for the fine grind required for espresso coffee-making equipment. An espresso-type roast is made from very oily, blackened beans. The taste of the carbonized cellulose usually overwhelms the natural aroma or flavor of the bean. Very intensely roasted robusta beans are often used, because the heat of roasting destroys the volatile flavor factors in better beans. In addition to the use of an inferior bean, the overroasting increases the acid-oils content. Both are suspected carcinogens, and both have been substantially indicted as stomach irritants.

Nor is it any coincidence that the term "espresso" is derived from the Italian word for "speed." According to the National Coffee Association, espresso has about twice the caffeine of 5.5 ounces of regular coffee, while instant espresso has slightly less caffeine than most popular instant coffees.[24]

That is no surprise, considering the fact that, customarily, two level tablespoons of drip- or fine-grind Italian-roast coffee are used for each demitasse cup.

Other Special Coffees

According to the San Francisco Consumer Action (SFCA), heavily advertised flavored "coffees," such as Suisse Mocha, Cafe Vienna, Orange Cappuccino, and Café Francais, are really coffee-flavored sugar and vegetable-fat solids, cleverly disguised by the addition of nearly a dozen artificial chemicals. And at $6.70 a pound compared to regular instant coffee at $4.70 a pound, that's a pretty steep price.

They are lower in caffeine for the simple reason that coffee constitutes less than 25% of the total. A typical analysis showed that these coffee treats were 53% sugar, 27% fat, and had ten artificial chemicals apiece.[25] Avoid them.

Coffee: Why We Drink It

Why do we do it? It gets us up, picks us up, keeps us alert, sobers us up, helps us lose weight.

The caffeine in coffee performs these acts by drugging the brain. According to researchers at the Johns Hopkins School of Medicine and at the National Institute of Arthritis, Metabolism and Digestive Diseases, caffeine affects behavior by counteracting the effects of adenosine in the brain. Adenosine normally inhibits the transmission of messages from one nerve cell to another and resembles a tranquilizer in slowing down brain and other body functions. In contrast, caffeine, which is structurally similar to adenosine, blocks this inhibition of nerve-message transmission by binding itself to the receptors normally occupied by adenosine, thus acting as a stimulant. But there's a price we pay for that lift.[26]

Energy, Coffee, and Alertness

Coffee has been called an amphetamine, or liquid speed. Two cups of coffee raise the metabolism 10 to 25%, the equivalent of 10 milligrams of amphetamine sulfate, which explains why amphetamine abusers are heavy users of caffeine pills.[27]

But the lift doesn't last. Caffeine saps energy. According to Dr. John Greden, former director of psychiatric research at Walter Reed Army Hospital, in some people even a few sips of coffee will elevate blood-sugar levels. In others, heart rate and blood pressure will increase. Capacity for muscular work may be temporarily stimulated, but since these effects are accompanied by nervousness and irritability, one hasn't really gained—one has lost.

What's more, increases in body function—such as the rise in blood pressure or heart rate—use energy. From an energy standpoint, nervousness and irritation only add to the daily burden of stress placed upon the body.

The lift one feels also unbalances the body's chemistry. And the body, recognizing the danger of elevated blood-sugar levels, sends insulin from the pancreas to drive the sugar level back down to normal. When too much insulin is produced, it results in low blood-sugar levels, and, with it, fatigue.

Age influences caffeine's effects, too. As another research study points out, "You get entirely different reactions to freshly brewed coffee from an elderly person and from a young, nervous person: The oxidation system of the elderly person is run down. He or she gets the sedative effect of caffeine and goes to sleep. The young, nervous person is a high-oxidizer and quickly changes the caffeine into trimethyl uric acid and feels like 'climbing the walls.' "

Using caffeine to stay alert at the wheel is unhealthy, too. In fact, Dr. Nelson Hendler, assistant professor of psychiatry at the Johns Hopkins School of Medicine, notes, "You're laying your life on the line if you depend on coffee to keep you alert and awake when you're driving. . . . About an hour after drinking coffee, your efficiency and alertness drop off. . . . The caffeine speeds up the heart rate and has an exciting effect on the brain, but within 30 minutes to an hour, the stimulation wears off and you 'crash' from your caffeine high. . . . If you speed up the release of brain chemicals far in excess of the brain's ability to produce more, you artificially excite until there's nothing left to excite."[28]

Sleep is another natural function affected by caffeine, especially at the levels found in coffee. According to researcher Charles Wetherall, brain-wave studies reveal that caffeine impairs the quality of sleep during the first three hours, when your metabolism is busy eliminating the caffeine taken in during the day.

Another study noted that caffeine also alters the quality of sleep. Far greater restlessness is exhibited by coffee drinkers who drink heavily. The heavier the intake, the more diminished the quality of the sleep.[29]

Caffeine users are frequently heavy barbiturate users. Both of these habits are among the stress factors that shorten life-span, sometimes by several years.

Coffee and Alcohol

Will caffeine undo what alcohol has done? Sometimes, sometimes not.

According to a study sponsored by the Insurance Institute for Highway Safety, if you've had a small to moderate amount of alcohol, less than three cups of coffee or the caffeine equivalent may help. But, adds the author of the study, Herbert Moskowitz, "If you've had a lot of alcohol, it won't work."[30]

And according to recent studies conducted separately by Britain's University of Hull and Indiana University's School of Medicine, volunteers who drank to the point of intoxication and then consumed two cups of regular coffee committed nearly twice as many errors in physical performance tests than drunk volunteers who didn't drink the coffee. "In no instance did caffeine counteract the alcohol—and in many cases it made it worse," says Dr. Robert Forney, distinguished professor of toxicology and head of Indiana's Department of Toxicology.[31]

Adds Benjamin Kissin in "Interactions of Ethyl Alcohol and Drugs," "Drinking strong coffee does nothing to make a drunken person less inebriated or to make him come around quicker. It's the level of alcohol in the blood that creates drunkenness, and there's nothing you can do."[32]

Coffee and Weight Loss

Dieters—that means one out of every four Americans—are big coffee drinkers. And coffee, after all, contains only five calories per cup.* As *New York Times* health reporter Jane E. Brody notes, "Coffee comes closer than any other part of the typical American diet to giving us something for nothing."

Does coffee actually help you lose weight? Yes and no. If you eat 2,000 calories a day and your weight is stable, then by stepping up your metabolic rate, "You start to lose a half-pound to a pound a week without even dieting," says Derek Miller, a leading researcher at the Department of Nutrition of the University of London. "And three cups of coffee or tea—without the extra calories of sugar or cream—increase it by 10 percent."

There are far better ways to step up your metabolism, of course. Exercise and a healthy pattern of low-calorie snacking throughout the day to keep blood-sugar levels stable are far better alternatives. It has been estimated that a good breakfast alone increases the metabolic rate by 14%.[34]

Filling your cup may fill you up temporarily without calories and take your mind off chocolate éclairs. But not for long. Coffee stimulates more than the central nervous system. It stimulates the appetite, and if you use cream, milk, or sugar in each cup of coffee, you could be adding thousands of calories a week, millions of calories a year, and be 10 to 15 pounds heavier at the year's end.

Even if coffee doesn't make you fatter, if it's an allergen

---

* Actually, 6 ounces of brewed black Maxwell House or Yuban contain only 2 calories. One cup of instant Sanka gives you 3 to 4 calories. Lowest of the low is a 6-ounce cup of regular or instant Chase and Sanborn. Either of these gives you what chemical analysis calls only a "trace" of calories.[33]

for you, it may make you look and feel fatter. According to Dr. James Braly, president of Optimum Health Labs, whose Encino, California–based firm specializes in cytotoxic testing, "Food allergens tend to cause fluid retention."[35]

Coffee beans are top-rated allergens (see Chapter 8). "Among the foods that frequently cause allergies and trigger the appetite are coffee, milk, soft drinks, chocolate, corn and chemical additives," says nutritionist H. L. Newbold.[36]

If you are allergically sensitive to coffee, milk, and the no-calorie chemical sweetener saccharin, and use all three, you could be in for considerable trouble.

What's worse, both instant coffee and instant tea contain corn, another of the top ten food allergens.

What about caffeine-containing diet pills? (See Table 15.) Forget them, is the best advice. The FDA's advisory panel may consider caffeine to be a safe ingredient in nonprescription diet pills at present, effective in fighting off the "well-known depressing effects of reducing diets," but it warns anyone using a combination pill to be careful about getting additional caffeine from other sources.

Each capsule or tablet contributes 100 to 300 extra milligrams of caffeine to your day's total. (See Tables 12–16.) If you pop a No-Doz (100 milligrams), take one caffeinated diet pill (200 milligrams), and knock off five cups of coffee, your caffeine total is nearly 1 gram. A lot, especially if your reducing diet isn't compensating for all the nutrients you're losing as a result of caffeine's diuretic effect.

An added problem is one of drug interactions. Most of these phenylpropanolamine and caffeine products are "fixed combination" drugs. And as Carol Ann Rinzler points out in her book *Strictly Female,* "If you are sensitive to caffeine or use it only rarely, some of the two-ingredient diet pills may perk you up so far that your friends will have to peel you off the ceiling. In fact, even if you are used to a couple of cups of coffee, tea, or cola every day, some phenylpropanolamine-plus-caffeine products can still give you quite a lift, both because of the amount of caffeine involved and because caffeine increases phenylpropanolamine's effects on blood pressure and pulse."[37]

Who knows what trouble you are asking for—and getting—if you are also on a doctor-prescribed medication as well?

We could quit if we wanted to—we've done it before. In 1950, coffee drinkers comprised 77.4% of the population. But by 1977, that figure had plunged to 57.9%, according to the International Coffee Organization. And by 1990, it is expected to hit a low of 16.7 gallons per capita.

The high price of coffee in 1976 and 1977, a result of a freeze in Brazil that damaged coffee trees, contributed to one of the first declines in consumption. The coffee industry says it has no idea how many people who stopped drinking coffee at that time never went back.

Unfortunately, if we're plugging in the percolator less often, it's only partly for health reasons. That consumption has been declining by 0.4% annually in recent years is true.[38] Price is another reason. And our continuing love of cola drinks is yet another.

The National Coffee Association admits caffeine's profile is lower than ever. As a result, coffee consumption declined almost 6.5% between 1970 and 1981. In 1975, for example, almost 20 million bags of green coffee were imported into this country, but by 1980, totals were down to 18 million bags.[39]

And what's taking coffee's place? Well, it isn't milk.

"Milk [is expected] to decline from its former lead position to per capita levels of 17.5 gallons by 1990.... Per capita consumption of coffee in 1960 was 35.7 gallons. In 1974, it declined to 24 gallons and is expected to decrease to 16.7 gallons by 1990.... Tea, with a nine percent growth rate since 1970, brought the per capita level to 12 gallons in 1979 ... should rise to 16.5 gallons by 1990.... Wines will experience their highest annual growth rate of eight percent.... And beer, in fourth position until 1979, will nose out milk and coffee for second place long before 1990."[40]

Recommendations

1. Quit or cut down to no more than two cups a day or switch to a caffeine-reduced "light" type of coffee, which has one-third the caffeine of brewed regular. Decaf is a better choice than regular, and grain coffee substitutes or herb teas are a better choice than most decafs.

2. Every extra minute of brewing time contributes extra caffeine. Six minutes is the maximum time to percolate; four to five is the limit for drip; and one to three minutes for vacuum brew and espresso-type machine.

3. Drinking coffee and smoking increases your risk of cardiovascular disease and, perhaps, cancer. Don't do both.

4. Drinking coffee or tea *after* a meal rather than with it or before it protects the lining of the stomach from coffee's irritation and from possible exposure to carcinogens enhanced by the presence of foods.

5. If you switch to instant coffee or regular tea to consume less caffeine, drink in moderation. Instant black coffee and tea both contain significant amounts of tannin, a substance that depletes vitamins, may cause constipation and stomach irritation, and may even damage the heart

37

muscle or cause cancer. (See section "Tannin, or Tannic Acid" in Chapter 4.) And remember, even decaf contains substances other than caffeine that disrupt normal brain activity and affect tranquility. (See Chapter 3.)

6. Buy a better bean to reduce your caffeine totals. Higher grown, better quality coffees have half the general caffeine (1.19 compared to 2.20%) of poorer quality brands, says the director of quality control for S. A. Schonbrunn & Co., a major coffee importer and processor.[41]

7. Learn to make a decent cup of coffee, and you'll drink less. The Coffee Brewing Institute has compiled a list of suggestions: (a) Buy a good-quality grind in small quantities. Coffee becomes stale within two weeks after being roasted, ground, and packed. Keep beans in a closed container in the freezer to prolong freshness for up to two months; it becomes stale in 90 days if packed in cans. (b) Start with a thoroughly clean coffee maker and use freshly drawn cold water. (c) Use the capacity of your coffee maker, and, for uniform results, consistent timing is important. Coffee should never be boiled (it concentrates caffeine). (d) Serve coffee as soon as possible after brewing. (e) Best results are obtained by using one standard coffee measure of coffee (or 2 level measuring tablespoons) to each 6 ounces of water. (f) Best material for pots are glass, ceramic, or stainless steel. And according to Robert C. Thomas of Manhattan's Coffee Brewing Center, "The person doesn't live who can make good coffee in an electric percolator. A Melitta or Melior pot is preferable, because it does not overextract or recirculate dissolved coffee solids."

8. One more hint from *The Pocket Guide to Coffees and Teas:* if you're buying roasted beans or freshly ground coffee, and the taste of a coffee is disappointing, the reason is likely to be that the beans are stale.[42] Never buy more than you can drink within a few weeks.

NOTE: The following tables do not list all the available national brands or types or products. And, of course, regional brands are excluded. Remember that formulations change. Read labels, consult your pharmacist, or write the manufacturer if you have questions.

Table 1. Caffeine Content of Coffee According
to Brewing Method

| | Percolator | | |
| | Nonelectric | | Automatic |
	5 min.	10 min.	
Regular coffee			
(5.5 oz.)	97–108	105–118	93–100
Average (mg.)	107	118	104

| | Drip coffee maker | |
	Nonelectric	Automatic
Regular coffee		
(5.5 oz.)	137–142	153–150
Average (mg.)	142	151

Table 2. Caffeine Content of Instant Coffee by Brand

Product	Mg. Caffeine per 5.5 oz.
Espresso (regular)	
Medaglia d'Oro	43
Spice Islands	55
Progresso	57
Reese	38
Blends	
Mellow Roast	30
Lite Reduced Caffeine	—
Luzianne	14
Freeze-dried	
Brown Gold 100% Colombian	66
Tasters' Choice	52
A&P Eight O'Clock	64
Maxim	62
Chock Full O'Nuts	53
Kroger	44
S&W 100% Colombian	52
Regular	
Nescafé	64
Maxwell House*	68
Spice Islands Antigua	56
A&P Bokar Premium Blend	43
Safeway	72
Yuban	65
Chock Full O'Nuts	53
A&P Eight O'Clock	41
Kroger Crystals	56
Hills Bros.	54
MJB	58
Savarin	63
Kava	68
Folger's Crystals	67

SOURCES: *Consumer Reports,* October 1979, and March 1983. Mary Louise Bunker and Margaret McWilliams, "Caffeine Content of Common Beverages," *Journal of the American Dietetic Association,* vol. 74 January 1979.

NOTE: Caffeine content of instant coffees generally ranges from 61 to 70 mg. per cup.

* The biggest-selling regular roasted, ground coffee.

Table 3. Caffeine Content of Decaffeinated Coffees

Brand	Type	Mg. caffeine per 5.5-oz. cup prepared as directed
Brewed		
A&P 97% caffeine free	Regular decaf	2
Nestlé Decaf	Regular decaf	2
High Point	Regular decaf	2
Sanka 97% caffeine free	Regular decaf	5
MJB	Regular decaf	1
Kroger Crystals	Regular decaf	1
Brim	Regular decaf	3
Brim	Electric perk	3
Sanka 95% caffeine free	Electric perk	3
Instant†		
Brim	Freeze-dried	2
Sanka 97% caffeine free	Freeze-dried	2
Taster's Choice	Freeze-dried	2
Sanka 97% caffeine free	Instant	2

SOURCE: *Consumer Reports,* October 1979. Manufacturers' data sheets, 1982.

† Instant decaf has about half the caffeine of brewed decaf.

Chapter 3

What You Need
to Know About
Decaffeinated Coffee

Is Sanka, America's best-selling brand of decaffeinated coffee, really "good coffee that makes good sense?" as spokesman Robert Young assures us? Is decaffeinated really the answer to your coffee-drinking problems? Don't count on it.

Consumption of regular coffee has been on a downswing almost continuously in the United States for the last 30 years. And this decline has been accompanied by a gradual though steady rise in the number of Americans drinking decaffeinated coffee.

Decaffeinated coffees are a $700 million market now.[1] Of the coffee sold in the United States in 1981, 20% was decaffeinated, a steep rise over previous years, and a 3% rise in 1980.[2] It's a change that's both good and bad.

In 1950 more than three-fourths of the population in the United States was drinking coffee (regular and decaffeinated) at a rate of 2.38 cups a person. By 1979 consumption had dropped to 57.2% of those over the age of 10 drinking at a rate of 2.06 cups a person.[3] The drop in consumption, the surveys indicated, occurred among *all* age groups, but primarily among those in the 10- to 29-year-old age group.

According to the New York–based National Coffee Association, 15% of the population drinks decaffeinated coffee at the rate of 2.4 cups a day per person (compared to 7.3% of the population drinking about the same amount in 1972). The decline of overall coffee drinking was "almost exclusively among those drinking regular coffee."

One of the top reasons for the switch, an industry spokesman noted, was the public's growing awareness and concern about caffeine consumption.

Decaffeinated coffee contains 2 to 15% (3% caffeine is average) of the world's most widely used drug. (The actual amount varies, depending on brewing time, type of roast, and type of grind. Instant decaf has about half the caffeine of regular brewed decaf.)

Rather than decreasing your risk of cancer and other diseases, switching to decaf may actually increase the risk. As bionutritionist Paavo Airola, author of the classic text *How To Get Well*[4] puts it: "It has not been conclusively proven what substance or substances in coffee are actually carcinogenic, or which of the substances is the worst carcinogen: caffeine, insecticides, acids, carcinogenic oils or tars and other toxic products developed during the roasting process. . . . Caffeine may not be the actual culprit at all; it may be the other substances in roasted coffee, such as tars, acids and natural oils subjected to extremely high roasting temperatures, that are the real carcinogens."[5]

If you are allergic to coffee beans, for example, you will be allergic to decaf. Since it is the beans, not the caffeine, that are the problem, removing caffeine doesn't remove the allergen. And if you drink it often, you run a higher risk of developing symptoms.

"When you eat the same foods day in and day out,

you increase the risk of developing an allergy to those foods," says Dr. Joseph McGovern, an adjunct professor at Brigham Young University currently involved in allergy research. "Possible symptoms include drowsiness, diarrhea, constipation, nausea, vomiting, migraine headache, hyperactivity, muscle pain, joint aches, hives and backache, mental depression and mood swings."

In 95% of food allergy cases, the reaction is caused by eating too much of a specific food. It is only in the remaining 5% that a person is born with an allergy, and eating patterns do not affect it.

More seriously, decaf has been cited as a causal factor in gastrointestinal disorders, peptic ulcer, cancer of the pancreas (pancreatic adenocarcinoma), myocardial infarction, and fibrocystic breast disease, which may increase the risk of breast cancer.

Decaffeinated beans may be just as great a source of toxins as regular coffee beans are. In addition, a recent abstract in the *Journal of Food Science* suggests that with the removal of caffeine during the decaffeination process, there may be an increase in the risk of contamination by one of the most potent carcinogenic substances now known—aflatoxin mold.

To start with, decaf is grounds for trouble even before it is processed. According to Frances Moore Lappe, director of the Food First Institute, "Pesticides, once dumped, come back to us like a boomerang, in our coffee. . . . Nearly half of the green coffee beans imported into this country are contaminated with pesticides that have previously been banned in the United States. . . . And that doesn't even take into account at least 20 pesticides, all potential carcinogens, that are undetectable with the FDA tests used to find residue in our food."[6]

Even after the caffeine is removed from coffee beans, a

few of the troublemakers still remain: ". . . substances such as sucrose, pectins, starch, hemicellulore, lignin, oils, protein, ash and acids such as chlorogenic, caffeic, quinic, oxalic, malic and tartaric."[7] There are other reasons why this deep-dark stuff spells trouble, even without caffeine.

According to a recent Harvard University study, if you drink decaffeinated or regular coffee, you may run an increased risk of pancreatic cancer. Investigators found that "habitual consumption of decaffeinated coffee was significantly greater among pancreatic cancer patients than controls." The finding presumably ruled out any link between caffeine and pancreatic cancer, because tea drinkers were included, and tea contains caffeine. The study noted that the chemical solvent tricholorethylene (TCE), widely used until 1975 to decaffeinate coffee, is the same chemical that was used to dry-clean clothes. The incidence of pancreatic cancer in the cleaning business is dramatically higher than in other professions surveyed.[8]

And Dr. Irving Kessler of the University of Maryland at Baltimore reported that 90.7% of patients with pancreatic cancer habitually drank decaffeinated coffee. In their case, regular coffee was not found to be associated with the malignancy, whereas decaffeinated coffee was.[9]

Methylene chloride, or dichloroethylene, the solvent in current use for decaffeinating coffee, has the same chemical structure as TCE, notes Emil Corwin, a spokesman for the FDA.[10]

Studies also indicate that between 40 and 50% of all coffee drinkers have gastrointestinal trouble. Although caffeinated coffee stimulates production of stomach acid, so does decaf, because it is the roasting of the coffee bean itself that releases harsh acids and oils that irritate stomach linings.

According to a report in the *New England Journal of*

Medicine, "The component responsible for the acid secretion may be a component of coffee other than caffeine.... Decaffeinization does not alleviate or lessen problems because acid secretion is only nominally reduced."

And a study by R. D. Paffenberger at the University of California at Berkeley of 25,000 men from college to middle age showed a 72% higher incidence of gastrointestinal complaints in those who drank coffee, *even decaffeinated,* than those who abstained.

Recently, experiments have been conducted to determine gastric-acid stimulation by regular and decaf coffee. Reporting in the *Journal of the American Medical Association* (July 17, 1981), a team of researchers at the Veterans' Administration confirmed previous studies. "Decaffeinated coffee," says Dr. Morton L. Grossman, "contains some unidentified ingredient that is a potent stimulant of gastric acid in man."[11]

And while regular coffee in excess of six cups a day raises your risk of heart attack by 50 to 100%, decaffeinated does a good job of it, too.

According to a study conducted with almost 13,000 patients in Boston-area hospitals, the risk of developing myocardial infarction (degeneration of the heart muscle) appeared just as high among drinkers of decaf as it did among regular coffee-drinkers.[12]

And although that 3% or so milligrams of caffeine in decaf may not seem like a lot, it's enough to cause other ills. According to Dr. Solomon Snyder, director of neuroscience at the Johns Hopkins School of Medicine, caffeine inhibits the action of a compound called adenosine, the building block of DNA that acts as a natural nerve depressant.[13] When you need to slow down, in other words, caffeine can keep the message from getting through.

According to Dr. John P. Minton of Ohio State University, who has done extensive research on methylxanthines (central nervous stimulants) and fibrocystic breast disease, drinks containing methylxanthines in *any* amount should be avoided. Major methylxanthine-containing beverages include regular and decaffeinated coffee and tea, cola, and pepper-type soft drinks, as well as chocolate and cocoa. Dr. Minton advises women with benign fibrocystic disease to stop consuming xanthine drinks, and has found that once caffeine and other methylated xanthines are eliminated, fibrocystic lumps usually disappear. In one of Dr. Minton's experiments, thirteen of twenty women with benign breast lumps experienced complete disappearance of all nodules and symptoms within 2 to 6 months of stopping consumption of caffeine. Only one in twenty-seven women continuing caffeine ingestion experienced complete recovery. And the younger the woman, the more likely it is that the lumps will respond to dietary changes.[14]

How are the chemicals in coffee and tea related to fibrocystic disease? It is speculated that the methylxanthines step up cell proliferation in fibrocystic tissue by prolonging the growth rate of fibrous tissues. The action of the methylxanthines interferes with certain tissue enzymes that would normally "turn off" the growth of certain tissues. Left to multiply at a faster than normal rate, the fibrous tissues grow into masses, which are usually surgically removed.

By themselves, says Minton and other researchers, fibrocystic growths are not usually cancerous, but women who develop such growths develop breast cancer at a rate four times higher than women who do not develop such growths.

Furthermore, research on Dr. Minton's findings indicate

that prostate problems could be connected with both regular and decaffeinated coffee drinking.[15]

The problem with a halfway measure like switching to decaf rather than switching off caffeine entirely is that the caffeine is only half of the problem. The other half, as already noted, relates to the chemicals used to remove the caffeine, and the chemicals with which coffee beans are treated.

Methylene chloride, the one currently used in removing caffeine, for example, says John Tobe, author of *Treasury of Natural Health Knowledge*, "is a solvent used for degreasing and cleaning fluids. It has been used as an inhalation anesthetic for minor operations, especially dental surgery. Its human toxicity is very high and may cause cardiac arrythmia, nausea and vomiting. It is obvious the food processors would be utterly derelict as to use such a deadly substance in a beverage used by millions of Americans."[16]

The *Journal of Norwegian Medical Associates* adds that "methylene chloride is a toxic gas used in the production of rubber, in paint remover, and as an anti-knock agent in gasoline."[17]

John Mennear, a toxicologist with the National Institute of Environmental Health Science, says that more test results on the solvent will be available soon.

The chemicals used to remove caffeine have always been unhealthy.* The first, benzene, used when decaffeination was introduced in the early 1900s, "is a potentially harmful cancer-causing chemical which can cause a variety of blood

---

* One that *isn't*, a pure water solvent process developed in Switzerland, has not been adopted by American firms, apparently because the chemical process is cheaper. Two brands are available in the United States: Rombout's from Belgium, and Cafix from Switzerland.

disorders, including leukemia. . . . It gets into the environment most commonly from auto and truck exhausts."[18]

And until 1975 the makers of Sanka and Brim were using trichloroethylene, a solvent in the same family as methylene chloride. Both chemicals are composed of chlorinated hydrocarbons, as are many widely used pesticides and insecticides. Trichlorethylene was used to degrease Sanka and Brim, both General Foods coffees. How were the carcinogenic effects of trichlorethylene discovered? By putting a gastric tube into the stomachs of mice and feeding them large amounts of trichlorethylene.[19]

In 1982 studies at the laboratories of the National Cancer Institute indicated that trichlorethylene could be carcinogenic. Tests made by the institute with trichlorethylene produced live tumors in the livers of 30% of mice, both male and female, fed low doses and 42% of mice fed high doses. The rats also developed tumors in their adrenal cortex and pancreas.[20] Sanka and Brim quickly switched to methylene chloride, presumably the less toxic of the two substances.

Although the initial research involves large doses of methylene chloride, still, there is, in fact, no proof that methylene chloride is safe. (According to spokesmen for the National Coffee Association, a person would have to drink 12 to 24 million cups of decaffeinated coffee a day to equal the amount of methylene chloride the research mice received.) The Health and Human Services toxicology unit has it under active investigation, and the FDA, with some caution, promises that its safety will be reviewed in the near future and that its status may change.[21]

Unfortunately, reports by researchers who have employed the Ames test, which measures carcinogenicity by mutation to growing salmonella cultures, show that meth-

49

ylene chloride is actually more mutagenic than tri-chlorethylene by perhaps two or three times.[22]

There are two stories about the origin of the decaffeina-tion process. According to the first, decaffeinated coffee probably resulted from an accident in 1900, when a ship-ment of beans headed for Germany was soaked by sea water coming through an open hatch. While trying to rid the coffee beans of salt, it was discovered that pressurized steam forced out the caffeine. A German chemist, pursuing the experiments further, discovered that some solvents, for example, chloroform and benzene, could *also* remove caf-feine from coffee beans and tea leaves.

According to the second story, decaffeinated coffee was born because a German entrepreneur became convinced that his father, a coffee merchant and taster, had died from an overdose of caffeine. It led the son, Dr. Ludwig Roselius, to patent in 1908 a process for decaffeinating the coffee bean. He founded his decaffeination operation, Kaffee H.A.G., in Bremen, Germany, and from the French, *sans caféine,* he named his coffee Sanka. He initially produced the coffee in Germany and France and then, just before World War I, started producing it in the United States. Eventually, *sans caféine* became the Sanka we know today.

Roselius's basic method was to heat the unroasted cof-fee beans with steam to raise their moisture level and then to extract the caffeine from the beans with a chemical sol-vent. The beans would be washed, steamed, and dried be-fore being roasted and ground for consumption.

Today, almost all manufacturers use this basic method, called the direct-contact method. In this method, coffee beans—in 5,000-pound batches—are placed in a large con-tainer and steamed to raise their moisture level to about 30 to 40%. This draws the caffeine to the surface of the bean. A chemical solvent is then poured into the kettle, drained, and recycled through the beans until 97% of the caffeine is removed. The process, to this point, takes about 12 to 18 hours. The solvent is then drained, steam is used to strip the residue of solvent, and the beans are then dried, roasted, and ground for consumption.

Because a small amount of solvent is left on the decaffeinated beans during the extraction process, FDA regulations state that the residue on coffee beans must not exceed ten parts per million. Most blends contain only about two parts per million, says the FDA.[23]

There are two safer ways to produce decaffeinated coffee, but not all manufacturers are using them—they are costly, and manufacturers are complacent.

One method, which has had FDA approval since January 1982—in response to a petition from General Foods—makes use of ethyl acetate. Also a common solvent, ethyl acetate has been used in Europe as a confectionery flavoring. So far, it appears safe for human consumption. In the body, ethyl acetate breaks up into two harmless chemicals—alcohol and acetic acid.

What chemicals are currently used to take the caffeine out of coffee? Chances are you won't have much luck in finding out. The coffee industry says it does not have this information. Nor does the FDA. Most aren't telling. However, in April 1983 the makers of High Point instant coffee—the Folger Coffee Company, a subsidiary of Procter & Gamble—disclosed they were removing caffeine with ethyl acetate because it is approved as safe and effective by the FDA. It occurs naturally in a number of foods, for example, apples, bananas, and pineapples. It is also approved by the FDA as a flavor ingredient and is used widely as such in a variety of foods and beverages. It has also been used as a decaffeinating agent for many years in Europe.[24] According to the Center for Science in the Public Interest, located in Washington, D.C., "Most other coffee producers including General Foods Sanka and Brim, Hills Brothers and Safeway Supermarket brands use methylene chloride."

Asked why all of America's decaf makers have not sought a chemical-free method, George Boecklin, president of the National Coffee Association, said, "I don't see why they should change. Methylene chloride has been approved for use by the FDA."[25]

The second method that is safer than methylene chloride, which *has* gone beyond the test-tube stage, is steam or water-process decaffeination.

It's easy to see how and why water-process decaffeination is preferable to all others. Although a solvent is still used, it never touches the bean itself. Instead, the raw beans are soaked in hot water, which leaches both oils and caffeine out of them. The solution is then removed to another chamber, where the solvent is added. The solvent combines with the caffeine and is separated out, leaving the purified solution. This solution is then put back into the chamber containing the beans, where the beans reabsorb the oils.

"But even these procedures," say researchers, "are still not completely effective at removing traces of solvent from the final product, but many drinkers think a better-tasting coffee is the result. Swiss and German companies developed the water process and are its main practitioners. For added cachet, some stores label their decaffeinated beans as "Swiss water-decaffeinated," but the important thing to note is that the water process was used."[26]

According to Robert Shedlock of the White Coffee Corporation in Long Island City, New York, which manufactures and distributes many coffees, only two companies—Cafix in Switzerland and Rombout's in Belgium—use the pure water method. Most European decaffeinators, he says, use methylene chloride just like those in the United States.[27] Both Cafix and Rombout's are available in health food stores, and others may also become available in the near future.

Recommendations

1. Switch to a water-extraction decaffeinated brand such as Rombout's. Another is available from health food stores, Café Hag, which uses no chemicals and calls itself Europe's premier decaf.

2. If you buy instant, switch to an acetate-decaf brand, such as Procter & Gamble's High Point or Maxwell House's Sanka.

3. Mix your decaf half and half with a grain coffee substitute that is coffee-bean-free, to reduce caffeine and other dangers. (Recipes appear on pages 173–177.)

4. You don't have to give up on quality completely if you quit caffeine. Reduce your overall intake, and just pick the best decaffeinated bean. Although the type of roasting has an important effect on the taste of the coffee, the origin of the bean is what determines true quality. A number of beans considered the most flavorful are also available in decaf form these days. Traditionally identified by location, these include Brazilian Santos, Colombian Manizales, Costa Rican, Yemen Mocha, Guatemalan Antigua, Haitian, Mocha-Java (a blend from Java and Yemen that does not contain chocolate), Hawaiian Kona, Jamaican Blue Mountain and High Mountain Supreme, Ankola, Tanzanian, Jalapa, and Ethiopian Harrar. (Note that decaf beans—whole or ground—unlike other regular beans, tend to change flavor, developing a faint caramelized taste. Don't buy more than a two-weeks' supply at a time, and refrigerate that.)

5. Look for as caffeine-free a bean as possible. Robusta beans are inferior in quality and generally contain *twice* as much caffeine as the arabica variety, meaning a decaffeinated robusta still contains 50% more caffeine than a decaffeinated arabica after 97% of the caffeine has been removed. Remember, too, that all decaffeinated coffees are not processed to remove 97% of the caffeine. Therefore, all decaffeinated coffees are not equally caffeine-free. Regular decaf has twice the caffeine of instant decaf (see Table 3).

6. See Chapter 10 for recipes and ideas.

Chapter 4

What You Need to Know About Tea

Tea. It's suited America to a T since 1650, the year it was first introduced in the Colonies. The year 1650 also saw the first tea imported commercially to England.

In 1660, a broadside advertisement by coffeehouse-owner Thomas Garway listed tea's virtues:

It maketh the body active and lusty.

It helpeth the Headache, giddiness, and heaviness thereof.

It removeth obstructions of the Spleen.

It (being prepared with milk and water) strengtheneth the inward parts, and prevents Consumptions, and powerfully assuageth the pain of the bowels.

It is good for Colds, Dropsies and Scurveys, if properly infused, purging the Blood by sweat and urine, and expelleth infection.[1]

One of the reasons tea does all that and more is that it contains not one but three of the central nervous stimulants known as the methylxanthines: caffeine, theophylline, and theobromine. It contains less than coffee, more than cocoa—and enough to cause problems. Six ounces of regular tea, according to the 1982 Michigan State University Data Base, contains about 67 milligrams of caffeine, while a one-cup serving of instant tea has about 27–30 milligrams.[2] It depends on the tea and who you talk to.

It is the presence of these stimulants plus two more naturally occurring troublemakers—oxalic acid and tannin—that makes tea seem a lot less cozy once you know they're there.

Excessive consumption of nonherbal tea can cause everything from migraine headaches to constipation, as well as deficiencies of the water-soluble B-complex and C vitamins, leading to iron-deficiency anemia, and even a mild form of beriberi, the B-1 (thiamine) vitamin-deficiency disease.

Heavy tea drinking can also shortchange you on protein and sleep, and may even be a factor in cancer. If you are a dedicated tea lover, you drink an average of 12 gallons a year. Fortunately, most of us in the United States are less than average tea drinkers. For most of this century, the annual tea consumption in the United States has ranged between ½ pound and 1⅕ pounds per person. In 1976 Americans consumed slightly less than 1 pound of tea per capita, enough to make about 160 6-ounce cups.

The United States imports only 160 million pounds of tea a year, enough to make 40 billion cups of moderately caffeinated cheer a year (a typical cup of tea has roughly 35 milligrams of caffeine, compared to coffee's 85). The English, Scotch, Welsh, and Irish tea lovers consume over 50% of the world's total tea output, averaging nine cups of tea for each cup of coffee. Canada averages 3 pounds per capita, and Australians and New Zealanders, 7 to 8 pounds. The highest consumption in Europe is said to be by the Dutch, who use 2 pounds per capita a year.[3]

In America, when it comes to a caffeine fix, our real cup of tea is still coffee. In fact, less than 5% of all coffee drinkers who quit switch to tea for a placebo pick-me-up (although one-third switch to a variety of herbal drinks, including herbal tea).[4]

Nevertheless, tea—50% of it brewed from bags—holds its own—running one-fourth as high as our national coffee intake at present.

For one thing, more fitness means more tea. According to the Fitness in America Study sponsored by The Perrier Company, sports-minded adults and very active adults report a 10 to 14% increase in their tea-drinking patterns "because of athletic participation," giving beer drinking, which in recent years has risen 11 to 15%, a run for the money.

And much of that hot stuff is being drunk cold. Of the tea sold in the United States today, 80% is iced, compared to 2% for iced coffee.[5] Sales of iced tea are rising by 2 to 3 million pounds a year, according to figures of the U.S. Department of Agriculture (November 1979).

One good sign? Twenty-five percent of all tea sold today is caffeine-free. And by 1990, predict some sources, the market for herbal tea may grow to some $500 million.[6]

Tea in History

India, with its 13,166 tea plantations, is the largest producer, consumer, and exporter of tea in the world today. It exports 484 million pounds a year, largely to Great Britain, Ireland, and the United States. By comparison, China now exports only 65 million pounds a year.[7]

Two million people in India are involved in tea's production, and the Indians themselves are avid if unconventional customers for their own product. "It has permeated society. The laborers drink it with salt; the rest, swimming in sugar," says British tea planter Chris Allen, who owns a tea estate in Hoogrijan, Upper Assam.

Exactly what is tea? The regular caffeine-containing tea that most of us drink comes from the dried leaf of an evergreen plant, a member of the camellia family. The seeds are obtained by allowing certain tea trees to grow until they reach a height of about 20 feet. During the blooming season, the tree is covered by small white sweet-smelling flowers from which fruit resembling hazelnuts develop.

There are over 3,000 varieties of tea plants, but only three types—black, green, or oolong. The grading classification and processing of tea is a complex business. But from the health seeker's standpoint, green tea is the healthiest, black the unhealthiest, and oolong somewhere in between. As a bonus, the teas lowest in caffeine are also lowest in tannin, the suspected carcinogen that occurs in various amounts in most tea leaves.

Tea is even older than coffee. Legend has it that more than a century and a half ago, a British army officer spotted indigenous tea growing wild in Assam, and his discovery led to a thriving British industry employing several thousand British tea planters.

Originally, the Chinese drank their tea mixed with salt, ginger, and sometimes onions, notes food writer James Trager.[8] The word "tea" comes from a Chinese ideogram that is pronounced "chah" (a pronunciation that traveled to India, Persia, Russia, and Japan) or "tay" (the pronunciation brought to Europe by way of the Dutch).

By the mid-eighteenth century, England was importing 1 million tons of tea annually. Tea did not become popular in Japan until the twelfth century. The Dutch East India

Company brought tea home to Europe in 1609, but the British East India Company, which Queen Elizabeth chartered in 1600, soon established a monopoly on tea.

The first tea plantations in the English Colonies appeared only in the middle 1800s.[9] And Anna, wife of the seventh Duke of Bedford, is said to have originated the institution of afternoon tea and cakes to provide sustenance during the long break between breakfast and an eight o'clock dinner.

How Tea Is Made

Leaves for all three kinds of tea are first withered by exposure to the sun or by heating in trays for eighteen to twenty-four hours, until they are pliable. Oolong teas are partially fermented before being dried. Teas are graded according to the age of the leaves used. Orange pekoe, which is made from the newest, youngest leaves and terminal buds (sometimes called flower pekoe), is the best grade. Lower-grade teas include the popular pekoes.

Tea bags date back to 1904. Legend has it that a tea merchant, Thomas Sullivan, sent samples of his various tea blends out to customers in little hand-sewn bags. Customers found they could brew the free tea just by putting the bag in a cup and pouring in boiling water. Numerous orders for tea in bags were placed, and the rest is history.

Iced tea dates to the same year. An English tea salesman, Richard Blechynden, at the St. Louis International Exposition, the same Louisiana Purchase Centennial celebration that gave the world ice cream cones, was in desperation at selling so little of his product to fair-goers. Because of the summer heat, he put a chunk of ice in the tea urn— and put iced tea on the map. He was helped partly because most cold drinks at the time were alcoholic, and the temperance movement was booming in the Midwest.

Next to water, tea is the most popular drink in the world.[10] But nutritionally it doesn't give water a run for its money. Water is rich in the basic minerals, such as calcium, and trace minerals, such as zinc and copper. Even when it's contaminated, water is caffeine-free.

However, a single cup of one popular brand of tea brewed for 5 minutes may contain up to 90 milligrams of caffeine—more than you get from two cola drinks, and enough of a drug dose to destroy 25% of your body's supply of vitamin B-1.[11]

This amount of caffeine is enough to cause or worsen pain. Studies indicate that cutting down your tea intake or eliminating it entirely may be the way to a more pain-proof body. According to Mary Jane Hungerford, Ph.D., a private practitioner of holistic psychotherapy in Santa Barbara, California, B vitamins are quickly destroyed both by the diuretic action of the caffeine in tea and by the tannins it contains. A heavy caffeine habit "definitely increases anxiety, which can, in turn, make any pain worse," she says. Cutting down on caffeine and increasing B-vitamin intake helps switch off pain.[12]

Tea's Stimulants

By the time coffee was discovered, tea was already widely used throughout Asia as a stimulant. Chinese legend relates that Daruma, a Zen Buddhist leader, dozed off during a nine-year meditation. When he awoke filled with remorse, he cut off his eyelids. From the earth where they landed, a shrub grew, and the drink brewed from its leaves was tea—a drink that could ward off sleep.

Tea wards off sleep because it contains caffeine—sometimes a lot more than you think. A cup of tea may provide anywhere from 10 to 90 milligrams of caffeine (see Tables 4–6), the average being 35 to 41 milligrams. That's about half the caffeine found in a cup of brewed coffee, and two-thirds that in instant coffee.

Some brands and varieties of tea are higher in caffeine, and brewing methods can boost methylxanthine content, too. According to Dr. Quentin Regestein, director of the sleep clinic at Peter Bent Brigham Hospital and Women's Hospital in Boston, if you are one of the 35 million Americans with insomnia, look to your tea intake.[13] If you are sensitive to caffeine, tea may have a "wake-up" effect on your body that persists as long as 20 hours. If you drink two cups of tea, the effect is the same as drinking one cup of brewed coffee or one and a half cups of instant coffee.

The caffeine content of unbrewed tea leaves is actually higher than the caffeine in coffee beans. But because of the contrasting nature of the two brewing processes, tea as a drink contains far less caffeine. Caffeine also varies with the age of the tea leaves. The older the leaf, the higher the content of caffeine and other xanthines—theophylline and theobromine. Caffeine content also depends on tea-leaf variety. According to Kenneth Anderson, author of *The Pocket Guide to Coffees and Teas,* black teas, such as India Black and African Black, and oolong varieties, generally have the highest content, with 3 to 4% caffeine per dry weight, while Chinese and Japanese green teas are lowest in caffeine—generally about 2 to 3% caffeine per dry weight; these types are also lowest in tannins (see page 65).

A blend may be a blockbuster, relatively speaking, if it uses more than one caffeine-rich variety. Examples are English Breakfast Tea or Irish Breakfast Tea. These may actually have more caffeine than regular instant coffee. (See complete listings in tables.)

How about the teas most of us buy off our supermarket shelves? One study of popular tea brands, conducted by Daniel S. Groisser of Mountainside Hospital in Montclair, N.J., found that "in every case, in every kind of brew—weak, medium and strong—Red Rose had the most caffeine, then Salada, then Lipton, then Tetley."[14]

He found that weak Red Rose tea had 45 milligrams of caffeine, while a strong brew had 90. Weak Salada tea had 25 milligrams of caffeine, while a strong brew had 78. Weak Lipton had 25 milligrams while a strong brew had 70. Weak Tetley had 18 milligrams while a strong brew had 70. (See Table 4.)

Among popular imported teas, Twinings English Breakfast in a weak tea-bag brew had 26 milligrams of caffeine, while the strong brew reached 107 mg. A Twinings Darjeeling in a tea bag had 30 milligrams in a weak brew and 91 milligrams in a strong brew.

The teas we usually buy aren't jasmine or oolong but so-called "broken-grade blends," which represent 80% of the total crop, and make a *dark,* strong tea. So, pinpointing actual caffeine content is difficult, if not impossible.

Purchased by agents of U.S. companies, tea-bag blends arrive in aluminum-foil-lined tea chests, and are placed in bonded warehouses, where they await approval by the U.S. Board of Tea Experts. In commercial tea-bag blends, some companies use up to 20 or more varieties in an attempt to maintain a constant quality.

Besides Caffeine: Other Hazards

Tea contains two other xanthines—theobromine, which may be present in substantial amounts in chocolate and cocoa products but occurs only in trace amounts in tea, and theophylline.

According to an industry study by Dr. Alan W. Burg, a senior biochemist at Arthur D. Little Company of Cambridge, Massachusetts, there is actually less than 0.3 milligram of theophylline in a cup of black leaf tea and only undetectable amounts in other teas and cocoa.[15] Other sources give slightly higher figures.

Theophylline is one of the most common ingredients in combination asthma medicines, such as Tedral and Marax, used to treat serious asthma conditions (see Chapter 7). But in large doses, like caffeine, its chemical cousin, it can cause serious side-effect illnesses of its own, reports *The Allergy Encyclopedia.*[16]

The side effects caused by too much theophylline are similar to those suffered by heavy coffee drinkers. All the methylxanthines are converted in the body to theophylline. "Irritation of the stomach or intestines, the most common side effects of methylxanthines, can lead to nausea and sometimes to abdominal cramping. Headache and vomiting are associated with excessive doses. Because [they] stimulate secretion of stomach acid, patients with ulcers of the stomach or intestines should be cautious about using them. Methylxanthines can also affect muscles, which prevent the contents of the stomach from returning to the esophagus through a valvelike mechanism known as the gastroesophageal sphincter, or the cardiac sphincter. Relaxation of this sphincter permits material to flow backward from the stomach into the esophagus."[17]

In smaller doses, even the trace amounts of theophylline in tea may be upsetting to the digestive tract. According to a Danish study conducted in 1981, when volunteers, 23 to 30 years of age, were permitted to follow their usual diet supplemented by copious quantities of tea, they all developed constipation and dehydration. The researchers attributed this to theophylline, which they said causes extracellular dehydration through the kidneys and a secondary increase in intestinal fluid absorption. It also slows down intestinal functions.[18]

Tannin, or Tannic Acid

Tea presents another problem that brewed coffee doesn't but instant coffee does. It contains tannin.

Tannin is the same substance used to tan leather. But it is also found in the bark of oak trees, in tea leaves, in red wine, in the skins of apples, plums, and grapes, and even in a few herbal teas. It is a substance that, along with caffeine, gives tea its characteristic flavor.

The U.S. National Academy of Sciences, in their manual *Toxicants Occurring Naturally in Foods,* has this to say about tannin: "The total acceptable daily intake for a man is 560 milligrams. This, however, is below the total intake of tannin by some persons, which may be of the order of 1,000 milligrams a day in coffee, tea, cocoa, etc." And 1,000 milligrams (1 gram) may be a total worth worrying about. It could be a factor in cancer.

Tannins are not xanthines, but "they are harmful to body tissues," says Dr. Julia F. Morton, a University of Miami researcher, who has documented an apparent link between gastric cancer and excessive intake of tannin-rich brews. "Peppermint tea, for example, contains tannin in the range from 6 to 12 percent."[19]

Also, recent studies by the U.S. Department of Health and Human Services indicate a close relationship between cancer of the esophagus and exposure to tannins in Chinese tea drunk black. (Adding milk or cream to tea, studies indicate, binds the tannin and makes it less harmful; lemon, however, has no effect on tannin.)[20]

Teas from Ceylon and India contain *more* tannin than Chinese black tea or Japanese green tea.

"In Japan, there are some fairly well-defined areas of the country with an exceptionally high rate of cancer of the esophagus," says Dr. Donald R. Germann.[21] Sponsored by a National Cancer Institute grant, Dr. Mitsuo Segi of the Aichi Cancer Center in Japan studied the situation and in April 1975 reported that the unusually high rate of cancer has to do with the local consumption of a mixture described as "tea gruel."

Tea gruel is made by packing tea leaves tightly into a cotton pouch, boiling the pouch in water, adding rice to the pouch, and boiling again. When done, the rice is a drinkable tea-flavored mush that is swallowed at temperatures near boiling. Similarly, in Colonial days, cooked tea leaves were salted, buttered, and eaten on bread, while the tea, boiled till it was strong and bitter, was drunk without sugar or milk.

"Other regional associations between tea drinking and cancer of the esophagus crop up in the medical literature," says Germann. "There's a high incidence of the disease in some parts of India where tea gruel is unknown but where tea is taken at extremely high temperatures."

Dr. Germann adds that the tannins are more reactive at high temperatures, and there is a theory that contact with extreme heat damages the lining of the esophagus, making it more vulnerable to possible carcinogenic influences, such as the tannin in the tea.

According to another study, conducted in 1979 in India, black instant coffee, because of its tannin, may be harmful to the heart and circulatory system. When rats were fed a diet rich in tannin, they experienced damage to their heart muscle and an increase in the cholesterol level of their blood. The rats received the human equivalent of six cups or more of black tea or black instant coffee per day. Both boiled loose leaf tea and instant coffee were found to be richer in tannin than regular percolated coffee and tea made from tea bags containing less of the acid. Adding one-fourth cup of milk to a cup of black coffee or tea reduced the tannin content by about 30%.[22]

Tannin and Nutrition

Robert McCaleb, a well-known biologist and a laboratory director at Celestial Seasonings, an herbal tea company in Boulder, Colorado, notes that tannins are known to combine with proteins to make them less available to the body and that they also inhibit the absorption of calcium and the B vitamins.[23]

According to Carol S. Farkas of the University of Waterloo in Ontario, Canada, the tannins in tea also combine with iron and prevent its absorption, especially when the diet is already inadequate.[24] The problem is greater when vitamin C is also deficient. Vitamin C and iron work together. Each is better absorbed in the presence of the other.[24] Research shows that high tannin intake at mealtimes may inhibit iron absorption from vegetable sources. Iron found in meat isn't affected.

Tannin-rich teas even bind the iron in the food supplements you take, possibly by forming insoluble iron tannate complexes. Vegetarians, therefore, with a heavy tea habit, are at a special risk, whether they take supplements or not.

A further problem, found by Dr. Germann, is that iron deficiencies have been linked with gastrointestinal cancers.[25] And according to studies done at the University of Kansas Medical Center, "The addition of tea to a meal previously measured for iron produced a drop of 64 percent in iron absorption. Coffee, which also exhibited an inhibitory effect, produced a drop of 39 percent. This study is important to pregnant women and all women of childbearing age where iron stores may be marginal to begin with." (This decrease in iron absorption can be offset by consuming tea along with vitamin C. A single glass of orange juice, containing 50 to 70 milligrams vitamin C, increases iron availability as much as threefold.)

According to experiments reported at a meeting of the Federation of American Societies for Experimental Biology in 1976, four to six cups of tea daily, even when used to wash down a well-balanced diet, can induce deficiency of the B vitamins.[26] Symptoms may include fatigue, nervousness, and loss of appetite. Within a week after beginning the tea-drinking regimen, all the volunteers in this study showed low thiamine levels, and "marginal to severe biochemical vitamin B1 deficiency." Scientists theorize that a chemical or physical union of the vitamin to the tannin in the tea made the vitamin unavailable.

Dr. Doris M. Hilker, an associate professor in the Department of Food and Nutritional Sciences at the University of Hawaii's College of Tropical Agriculture, agrees. Studies revealed that the heavy consumption of tea—one quart a day— can reduce one's level of the vitamin B-1 by as much as 60%.

According to Dr. Hilker, "When people have a vitamin B1 deficiency, they become tired, nervous . . . they have a general malaise, aches and pains—particularly at night. . . . This progresses to a kind of tingling in the legs, the feet . . . then it goes on to cardiovascular disturbances, lack of appetite, and it can proceed to death. It can kill you if you have a serious thiamine deficiency. . . . Right now, we don't know which drink is worse: coffee or tea."

If you sweeten your tea with lots of sugar, you have double trouble, because vitamin B-1 is then depleted even faster. Half a milligram of thiamine is needed to "burn" 1,000 calories. Since neither sugar nor tea supply B-1, a diet rich in sugary tea, even though adequate in vitamin B-1, can (and does) produce "clinical symptoms of thiamine deficiency, including many alterations of behavior ordinarily attributed to severe neurosis."[27]

To complicate matters, tannins in tea can interact with ingested medications—especially drugs that are alkaline in nature, such as painkillers, antihistamines, and tranquilizers—and prevent their absorption. Adding cream or milk to the tea helps neutralize some of tannin's harmful effects, as noted previously.[28]

Tea—Good News and Bad News

Are there any health benefits to be derived from tea? A few.

If you suffer from a form of hereditary anemia known as thalassemia, or sickle cell disease, you absorb too much iron. The tannin-containing tea might be helpful.[29]

Also, according to studies by the Department of Microbiology at the School of Dental Medicine at Washington University in St. Louis, Missouri, teas high in fluoride have been shown to reduce dental decay by as much as 60% by strengthening calcium in the teeth.

High-fluoride teas and the daily amounts required for a calcium-strengthening effect include ten cups of instant or Ceylonese tea, five cups of domestic black or black blended tea (including decaffeinated), one and a half cups of China black tea, one cup of green or Russian tea, and a half cup of oolong tea. The teas should be steeped for 3 minutes in a covered pot to obtain maximum results.[30]

All in all, tea is considerably safer than coffee, even if it doesn't get a clean bill of health.

One reason for its comparative safety is that most tea drinking is done at a level of one to two cups daily—three to four, at most. Few of us consume eight, ten, or fifteen cups of tea a day, something millions of coffee drinkers do without a second thought.

Second, the caffeine level of brewed tea is lower than that of coffee. A cup of tea with 60 milligrams of caffeine is considered to have a high level of the substance; most teas only contain 35 milligrams per cup, with an average of 40 milligrams (green teas average 27 milligrams of caffeine per cup, compared to 125 milligrams of caffeine for coffee). Obviously, your central nervous system benefits by this reduction.

Nor does tea contain quite the collection of hazardous oils and acids found in both regular and decaffeinated coffees.

Another reason is that, as researcher Charles Wetherall points out, "The caffeine content of teas has remained largely the same over history. Teas have not been subject to the insanity of mass market blending that has gone on so ruthlessly in the coffee business—particularly in the past 20 years. And it's that 'special' blending that has caused so many of our caffeine troubles."[31]

Decaf Teas vs. Herbal Teas

Are the new 97% decaffeinated teas the answer? Yes and no. Since they only contain 3% caffeine, such teas are healthier. But a further problem exists. Why haven't more tea marketers entered the field? "The difficulty is in patenting a flavorful extracting process," says a Lipton Company spokesman, "that is flavorful but chemical-free."*

"We continue to look at decaffeinated teas, but frankly find the chemical process unacceptable," says Celestial Seasonings, the country's largest herbal tea maker. "Plus, we don't feel anybody has really perfected a decaffeinating process that keeps the real tea flavor. We plan to resist the temptation until we can brew a decaf that is chemical-free."[32]

Recommendations

1. Learn to make a proper pot of tea, and you'll use less tea and consume less caffeine and tannin. According to the London Tea Council, here's how:

- Always use fresh cold tap water. Hot tap water or water that has been left standing in the kettle will be flat and without the oxygen content that gives tea its sprightly flavor.
- Heat the teapot with scalding water, and do not empty it until just before brewing time. Leaves should not sit in a damp pot for more than a second before they are covered with boiling water, or they will develop a stewy, burnt vegetable taste.
- The best proportion for brewing is one scant teaspoonful of leaves for a 5.5-ounce cup of water. An extra teaspoonful for the pot? It's a traditional custom you can skip.
- Bring water to a rolling boil in a kettle, then pour it

* In the spring of 1983, Lipton became the first tea maker to introduce a decaffeinated version of its regular tea. Bigelow (manufacturer of the popular "Constant Comment") also offers decaffeinated versions of its most popular brands. Check supermarket shelves and your local health food store for others.

over the leaves. Allow 3 to 5 minutes for brewing. No more. Stir or swirl leaves to release more flavor.

- Taste, not color, is what determines proper strength, although color can be a guide to tannin. Leaves brewed longer than 5 minutes release extra tannin and give an unpleasantly dry, acidic flavor to the brew.
- For a weaker brew, use fewer tea leaves.
- Serve tea immediately—never reheat. Reheating increases the concentration of caffeine.

What else? Don't use metal spoons and metal infusers. They interfere with tea flavor, because plant alkaloids are sensitive to metallic ions. A ceramic pot, or a bamboo strainer, is better.*

2. Switch to a safer tea, preferably herbal or at least decaffeinated. Supermarkets now carry such teas. (See Chapter 10 for more tea you can make and buy.)

3. There are countless different kinds of flowers and herbs that are stimulant-free. Hayfever sufferers should avoid, in general, teas made from the flavor heads of marigold, goldenrod, chamomile, yarrow, and chrysanthemum. Teas made from *yerba maté,* passion flower, and *kava-kava,* as well as Mormon tea, contain noncaffeine stimulants. But the virtues of ginseng and *gotu kola* probably outweigh the negative fact that they also contain noncaffeine stimulants.

Gotu kola, for example, which is called Chinese violets in Hawaii, has been used throughout history as a tonic for the system and as a heart stimulant by the Indians, Hawaiians, and Japanese. Indian authorities assert its usefulness in diseases of the nervous system, in memory improvement, and in the treatment of leprosy lesions and symptoms.[33]

* Or write to Anne Ross, inventor of Le Tea Baguette, a do-it-yourself teabag kit—Box 47, Fort George Station, New York, New York 10040.

Herbal teas are generally brewed the same way as regular tea. Use two teaspoons per cup of boiling water. If fresh herbs are used, double the quantity. Herbal teas can be vitamin-fortified by combining them with fresh fruit juices. Serve them plain, or flavor them with powdered fruit rind, honey, or lemon juice.

A few good herbal teas to try for starters include (a) dried leaf types, such as alfalfa, blueberry, parsley, mint, and comfrey; (b) dried blossom types, such as clover, linden, and chamomile; and (c) dried berries, or seed types, such as rose hips, alfalfa, anise, and dill. Avoid licorice root, which can be toxic in large amounts, and sassafras, which is a suspected carcinogen.

4. If you've kicked the coffee habit, put your automatic drip coffee maker to good use. Use it to brew herbal tea, economically and by the potful. Place the paper filter in the basket, and add loose herbal tea. You could also use tea bags, but the idea here is to save money. Pour water into the reservoir and brew delicious, inexpensive herbal tea in minutes.

5. To avoid excessive tannins, let tea color be a tip-off. The darker the tea, the likelier it is to contain lots of tannin. Light-colored herbal teas, such as linden or chamomile, are both tannin-free and caffeine-free. But teas brewed from wax myrtle leaves, sweet gum tree leaves, and the root of marsh rosemary all contain tannin. Chinese and Japanese teas generally contain less tannin than black imported teas. In general, most teas high in caffeine are rich in tannin, too. And drink your tea warm, not hot. Tannins become *more* carcinogenic at high temperatures.[34]

6. Never use tea to wash down medications or vitamin C. The tannins in tea reduce their effectiveness.[35] And remember, adding milk or cream helps neutralize some of the harmful effects of tannins. But don't oversweeten. Sugar destroys the B vitamins, numbs the palate, and stimulates the appetite, leading to second cups.

7. See Chapter 10 for more hints and product information.

NOTE: The following tables do not list all the available national brands or types of products. And, of course, regional brands are excluded. Remember that formulations change. Read labels, consult your pharmacist, or write the manufacturer if you have questions.

Table 4. Caffeine Content of Teas

	Mg. per 5-oz. cup		
Product	Weak brew	Medium brew	Strong brew
Brand			
Red Rose	45	62	90
Salada	25	60	78
Lipton regular	25	53	70
Tetley	18	48	70
Twinings English Breakfast			
tea bag	26	78	107
loose	39	—	90
Twinings Darjeeling (tea bag)	30	74	91
Jackson Formosa (loose)	42	—	78

Iced Tea (12-oz. can)   22 to 36 mg
Instant Tea (per cup)   45 mg

NOTES: These are averages. The brew could be 6 to 7% higher or lower, depending on brand. In general, loose tea averages about 35 mg. per cup; instant tea, 24 mg.

There is approximately 1 mg. or less of the caffeine-related stimulant theophylline in most teas, although it may reach 6 mg. in some brands of instant tea.

Theobromine content ranges from 2 mg. to 9 mg. in most teas.

Table 5. Caffeine Content in Tea*

| | Average caffeine per 5-oz cup | | |
Type	Weak (2 min.)	Medium (3 min.)	Strong (5 min.)
Black bagged tea	28	42	46
Green bagged tea	14	27	31

SOURCES: *Tea and Coffee Trade Journal.* January 1975. *Consumer Reports,* October 1981. *American Journal of Clinical Nutrition,* vol. 31, pp. 10–78. *International Journal for Vitamins and Nutrition Research,* vol. 46, 1976. *Better Nutrition,* February 1979. Wisconsin Alumni Research Foundation, 1976 Analysis. Madison, Wis.

NOTES: Green teas do not undergo oxidation. They remain green and produce a milder brew lower in caffeine and tannin. Oriental teas, in general, are safe.

Black teas undergo a special process of oxidation (fermentation) that turns them black and produces a strong brew. They are higher in caffeine and tannins and are used mostly in Western nations, including the United States. Some of the better-known varieties are Assam (India), Darjeeling (India), Keemun (China), Lapsong Souchong (China), Earl Grey (blend), and English Breakfast (blend).

Oolong-type teas are semioxidized (fermented). Examples include Taiwan oolong and jasmine.

* Formulations are subject to change.

Table 6. Herbal Teas That Contain Caffeine

Tea	Description
Guarana	Made from seeds of Brazilian plant. Also sold in food stores as a "vitamin energy supplement" under various brand names including "ZOOM." Contains about triple the caffeine of brewed coffee.
Gotu kola	Sold as tea and supplement.
Yopo	Similar to *guarana*. Derived from tropical tree bark. Contains 1½ times caffeine of regular coffee.

Table 6. (Continued)

Tea	Description
Morning Thunder	Usually sold as herbal tea, but is a blend of two caffeinated teas—black tea and South American *maté*. Said to be 33% higher in caffeine than instant coffee. Product of Celestial Seasonings Co.
New Brazilian Breakfast	Blend from Celestial Seasonings. Moderate amounts of caffeine supplied by the *maté* it contains. *Not* an herbal tea.
Emperor's Choice	Product of Celestial Seasonings. Original contains 20% caffeine of black tea. There is decaffeinated version.
Maté (also *yerba maté* or Paraguay tea)	Derived from *Ilex* plant grown in Brazil and throughout tropics. Rivals coffee and tea for popularity throughout South America.
Cassina (also *yaupon,* Christmas berry tree, or North American tea plant)	Once common source of caffeine beverage among American Indians. During World War I, sold as coffee substitute. *Cassina*-flavored ice cream, soft drinks, and teas also marketed. Letting leaves of *cassina* ferment produces drink containing both alcohol and caffeine.

SOURCES: *Health Foods Business,* June 1980. Kenneth Anderson, *The Pocket Guide to Coffees and Teas* (New York: Perigee Books, 1982).

NOTE: All regular teas contain tannin, which is not a xanthine, but is a suspected carcinogen. Adding milk or cream to tea makes the tannins less harmful. (See page 66.) Ceylon, Indian, and black bone-leaf tea have the most tannin. Light Japanese and Chinese teas and tea in bags have the least tannin. Most herbal teas are tannin-free, with the exception of peppermint (6 to 12% by weight), root of marshmallow, rosemary tea, wax myrtle leaf, and sweet gum tree leaf.

Chapter 5

What You Need
to Know About Soda Pop

"A young child who drinks one cola may experience the same problems—irritability, irregular heartbeats, insomnia—as does an adult who has four cups of coffee," says Dr. Tom Ferguson, editor of the periodical *Medical Self Care*. But an adult who has four cups of coffee isn't likely to care whether his child has one Coca-Cola. After all, "Coke is it," as the slogan goes. But then, so is any *other* kind of soda pop that contains caffeine.

Four out of the six corporations that make their money on soda pop do it with cola-type drinks containing caffeine. Eight out of the ten of the soda pops that are top sellers are caffeinated with 45 milligrams of caffeine per can.

Sixty-two percent of the soft drinks sold in the United States contain caffeine—anywhere from 2 milligrams a can (Cragmont) to 60 milligrams (sugar-free Mr. Pibb).[1] If you're a caffeine drunk, Coca-Cola, the original, is a lesser upper among the uppers, as is Pepsi-Cola.

The average man, woman, and child in the United States drinks nearly 40 gallons of soft drinks per year. Soft drinks account for 35% of the United States beverage dollar. (Alcoholic beverages and milk account for 25% and coffee, for 20%.)

Soft drinks account for 8% of the calories consumed daily by the average person—a love affair we share with the rest of the world. At any given moment of any given day, 138,000 people throughout the world are having a Coca-Cola. The 1982 revenues for the corporate giant were $6.2 billion.[2]

Ironically enough, coffee drinking is what supports our cola habit. Most of the 2 million pounds of caffeine extracted from the beans used for decaf each year are purchased by the soft-drink industry.[3] Cola and pepper-type soft drinks account for 60% of the caffeine that is used in the United States food supply today.[4]

Soft drinks now outsell coffee, tea, and milk in the United States. Next to water, soda pop is America's favorite thirst quencher.[5] And soda pop with a kick in the can, in particular, is the pop we opt for the most.*

Put another way, if all the Coca-Cola ever produced was divided up among all the inhabitants of the world today, every person would get eleven cases, each case containing twenty-four bottles of the stuff. The world's most popular soft drink is advertised in eighty different languages, and people throughout the world consume 12.5 million gallons of it daily.[6]

That's just Coca-Cola. Other caffeinated soft-drink leaders, such as Dr. Pepper, aren't far behind. The soft-drink business is a $2.5 billion a year industry, and growing annually at a rate of about 3 to 4%.[7] The largest growth of all is in caffeinated sodas, especially colas.[8]

* Soft drinks have been outselling coffee, which *used* to be number one, since 1971. It is said that by the year 2014, soft drinks will have replaced even water.

Ranked by millions of cases shipped in 1982, the leaders are Tab (237), Diet Pepsi (180), Sugar Free Dr. Pepper (81.5), Diet 7-Up (79), and Diet Rite Cola (35).[9]

Who drinks cola? Who doesn't? There has been a three-fold increase in overall soda consumption since 1960. It's no longer unusual to find infants weaned from baby formula to soda pop reports one study, which showed that 40% of one- and two-year-olds consume an average 9 ounces of soft drinks a day. The caffeine intake ranged from 31 to 46 milligrams. (A cup of percolated coffee contains 110 milligrams of caffeine.)

Your son, on the other hand, probably did *more* than his share. Teen-age boys polish off an average of 22 ounces a day, whereas kids of all ages guzzle $8 billion worth of soda a year.[10]

In 1849, there were only 64 bottling plants to service the entire country. By 1910, the Coca-Cola Company alone had 379 plants. Today, there are 20 million machines vending caffeinated drinks, and Coca-Cola alone has cornered 80% of the 200,000 fast-food outlets.[11]

Consumption of soft drinks has risen 157% since 1900. Sales increased 50% between 1970 and 1979 alone.[12]

We drink almost 40 gallons of soda pop a year. By comparison Americans consume an average of 27.8 gallons of coffee a year, and milk is at a low of 24.8 gallons per capita.

In the United States, three caffeinated sodas have dominated almost two-thirds of the market for decades. While Coca-Cola controls roughly 26.6% of the soft-drink market, Pepsi has 19.5%, and Dr. Pepper holds about 7%.[13]

Sales of 7-Up, which is a just-as-available thirst quencher—and a lot less hazardous to health than colas—represented less than 7% of soft drink sales in 1982, while Coca-Cola and Pepsi combined got 54% of our business. As long as you're an "un-cola," it seems—you'll never be number one. Popular soft drinks without caffeine can provide other hazardous additives. 7-Up, which runs third behind Coke and Pepsi in market share, for example, "boasts" no artificial color or flavor, but it contains both citric acid, a preservative, and sodium nitrate, a chemical that converts into the carcinogenic substance nitrosamine.[14]

Added Caffeine vs. Natural Caffeine

The caffeinated pause that refreshes is almost a century old. It did more than refresh in the 1890s, when it first appeared. When you ordered a Coke, you really *were* getting the real thing. Coca-Cola's original formula, at least until the government stepped in, in 1902, contained real cocaine.

The original Coca-Cola was invented in 1886 as a nerve and brain tonic. Georgia pharmacist "Doc" Pemberton's original Coca-Cola syrup was a boiled mixture of extracts from kola nuts, untreated coca leaf, and fruit syrup. He first sold his syrup to Jacob's Drug Store in Atlanta. It was here that Coca-Cola got its name. The accidental addition of soda water changed the flat medicine into a pick-me-up. Twenty-five gallons of syrup were sold the first year, for a total of fifty dollars.

Advertising claimed that Coca-Cola "relieves mental or physical exhaustion, offering relief from biliousness (sluggish liver), indigestion, and nervous headaches." The combination of the coca leaf's anesthetic effect on the stomach, reducing hunger pangs, and the kola nut's reputation as a water purifier, strengthener, hangover cure, and "love potion" is what did it, says Lawrence Dietz in his book *Soda Pop.*[15]

America's concern about the long-term use of patent medicines and opiates resulted in the 1906 Food and Drug Act. And the Coca-Cola Company responded by removing the minute amounts of cocaine (known for its stimulating effects on the nervous system) from each coca leaf.

Sales for the Coca-Cola Company, almost a century later, hit the $600 million mark. In 1979, worldwide sales averaged 21 billion gallons.

The exact formula for Coca-Cola's syrup, known in the trade as 7X, is a closely guarded secret to this day. According to Taylor Quinn, acting associate director for compliance of the FDA's Bureau of Foods, "We know pretty much what Coke is—it's a kola nut extractive and the coca berry. It's precisely how much of each they add which is the big secret."*

But colas aren't the only soft-drink sources of caffeine. Caffeine goes into pepper-type drinks and some citrus sodas. It says so on the label.

But how many of us know that the one brand you wouldn't hesitate to give your child may contain more caffeine than regular tea? Or that 12 ounces of Mountain Dew soda has 25% more caffeine than regular Coca-Cola, while Sunkist soda has no caffeine at all?

According to the law, caffeine is considered Generally Recognized As Safe (GRAS) for use in certain nonalcoholic carbonated beverages† (soft drinks); in cola-type beverages, up to 0.02% is acceptable. (Caffeine occurs naturally in tea, coffee, and *maté* leaves, as well as in kola nuts.)

Under the government's Standards of Identity for Nonalcoholic Carbonated Beverages, caffeine may be added as

---

* Author E. J. Kahn, Jr., was refused any details of the formula when he researched the history of Coca-Cola for his book *The Big Drink*. "As near as I could figure out there were at least 14 things in their syrup, such as sugar, caramel, caffeine, phosphoric acid and a blend of three parts coca and one part cola," said Kahn,

† According to Consumers Union, caffeine levels as low as 0.01% of a soft drink can cause behavioral changes in some children.[16]

an optional ingredient; its presence must be stated on the label. Cola-drink manufacturers, however, successfully pressured the FDA to allow them the special privilege of avoiding this label declaration. Thus, although Federal law demands that cola drinks must contain caffeine, label declaration is not mandatory.[16] The *only* 100% caffeine-free cola available as of the summer of 1983? Caffeine-free Coke.

Why are the others, such as The Seven-Up Co.'s Like and Pepsico Inc.'s Pepsi Free only 99 percent? Because of the Food and Drug Administration's profile of a cola. It specifies, among other things, that a cola contains caffeine. So the caffeine-free products leave in a trace of caffeine for the right to be called a cola.

But the people at the Coca-Cola Company waived that right. The caffeine-free Coke label will read "carbonated beverage." The company hopes the extra percentage point will give it an edge in a market now crowded with 17 major cola brands, including six of its own, reports Jesse Meyers, editor and publisher of the *Beverage Digest* newsletter.

The irony of the entire caffeine-free situation? The FDA that mandated caffeine content in the 1930s (when it realized that the processing of kola nuts robbed the nuts of their natural caffeine), is the same one that in 1978 warned us of its possible deleterious effects.[17]

What's worse is that soda from soda fountains may be even more caffeinated than soda in cans. "Fountain syrups, in most instances, are formulated to produce a finished product in a 1:5 ratio," says *The Complete Junk Food Book*. "That is, one ounce of syrup for every five ounces of water equals six ounces of soda. Accordingly, one gallon of 1:5 syrup will turn out 128 six-ounce drinks or 768 ounces of finished product which should have roughly 3 to 4 ounces of caffeine per ounce but may have much more. . . .

But it is virtually impossible to prepare the exacting proportions of water and flavored syrup required to make a satisfactory beverage at a fountain." In other words, it's possible to get Coca-Cola that's twice as caffeinated as it's supposed to be.

In 1978, caffeine was demoted from a 1 to a 3 on the government's GRAS list of food additives (GRAS 3 status means more tests are needed soon) in response to a report from the Federation of American Societies for Experimental Biology, concluding that "it is inappropriate to include caffeine among the substances generally recognized as safe. At current levels of consumption of cola-type beverages, the dose of caffeine can approximate that known to induce such pharmacological effects as central-nervous-system stimulation."

As a result, the FDA is proposing to make caffeine an optional ingredient, rather than a required one, in cola and pepper beverages, and to delete caffeine from the GRAS list. Instead, caffeine would be regulated as an interim food additive while the industry conducts mandatory research to resolve safety questions. Either way, there would be little effect on the public's exposure to caffeine.

Soft-drink manufacturers are already permitted to market cola and pepper beverages with as little caffeine as they want. They are not required to add caffeine, and they have the option to exclude almost all of it now. Cragmont Cola, sold in supermarkets in many parts of the country, has only 2%. And diet colas, such as RC100, needn't add caffeine at all because they come under a different FDA standard.

Secondly, the new "interim" status proposed for caffeine would have little practical effect, at least for several years. Deleting caffeine from the GRAS list means that manufacturers may not develop new uses for caffeine at will. But it could still be used in the food and drink to which it is currently added. Major safety questions could easily take many years to resolve.

Why Added Caffeine?

More than 95% of the caffeine in a typical cola or pepper beverage is added by the manufacturer. So is 100% of the caffeine in citrus-flavored soft drinks.

The question is if a cola drink already has kola nut extract in it, why does it need *added* caffeine? (Michael Jacobson of Washington's Center for Science in the Public Interest, in a report in 1980, suggested that unscrupulous manufacturers might some day add caffeine or other common psychoactive chemicals to a variety of foods to promote brand loyalty.)[18]

In Africa, the West Indies, Brazil, and India, where the kola tree grows, people still chew the nut itself for the "lift" from the caffeine it contains (about 2%). The kola nuts shipped to other countries are used almost exclusively in making cola soft drinks to impart a characteristic flavor and to give the usual "lift."

But the lift would be nearly as high without that *added caffeine*. Manufacturers say caffeine is there for the cola taste and to cut down the syrupy aftertaste.[19] But it's good for business, too. Of the best-selling soft drinks, Coca-Cola outsells caffeine-free 7-Up by a margin of over 500 million cases a year.

However, Consumers Union says that caffeine serves no uniquely essential function in soda. It also says that cola drinks can be made with decaffeinated kola nut extract, and safer additives might be found to cut the syrupy aftertaste as well as caffeine reportedly does.[20]

Caffeine is what manufacturers call a bittering agent.

Cola manufacturers say they add the bitterness of caffeine to colas to help offset their sweetness. But a spokesman for America's largest supermarket retailer—Safeway Stores, Inc.—suggests, "If there's such a thing as caffeine addiction, that may be why they do it."

"The American consumer is in love with the cola taste," said Lawrence Adelman, first vice-president of the investment company Dean Witter Reynolds.

Is it the taste or is it the caffeine that makes us drink more colas than noncolas? It may be no coincidence that the only noncola brands that have dramatically increased their share of the market in recent years are Pepsico's Mountain Dew, Coca-Cola's Mello Yello, and Dr. Pepper, all caffeinated noncolas.[21]

Yet, results of blind taste tests the Safeway Corporation conducted indicate that consumers cannot tell the difference between regular cola and Safeway's low-caffeine Cragmont soda, which uses decaffeinated kola nut extract.

These results could be useful to the FDA, which is considering a proposal to ban caffeine in soft drinks.

Who Provides the Biggest Kick

"Body by Tab" reads the ad, but maybe that's a label you'd rather not wear.

What's missing in Tab that you get from Coca-Cola is the calorie equivalent of nine teaspoons of refined sugar. It adds up.

The average user of diet cola* "typically consumes 1,839 calories daily—11 percent less than the 2,055 calories consumed by the average person who drinks nondiet beverages."[22]

* Diet sodas account for 10% of all soft drink sales.

But to make up for the missing stimulation and flavor of sugar in diet sodas, processors often add 2 to 10% *more* caffeine to diet sodas than to regular caffeine-containing sodas, with the exception of Mountain Dew, Mello Yello, and Diet Mr. Pibb, which *are* higher in caffeine. Mello Yello also uses BVOs (brominated vegetable oils) in its formulas.

But is it worth the risk for a few saved calories?

Tab and the other diet colas, in addition to caffeine, which is suspected as a carcinogenic catalyst, also contain saccharin or a sugar substitute that is an acknowledged carcinogen. (See pages 130–131.) According to the government's Food and Nutrition Board, more than four diet sodas a day is unadvisedly "heavy" for an adult.[23]

Table 7 lists the amount of saccharin and caffeine you got in 1981 from various popular diet colas:*

By contrast, noncola-type diet sodas contain *no* caffeine, and they contain less saccharin. See, for example, Table 8.

See Table 10 for complete listings of various soft drinks.

The Hazards

Only 3.2% of the over-18 population indulges in cocaine.† But 55% of us have a Coca-Cola habit. And a large percentage of these users are children.

Cocaine and caffeine both cause the nerve center in the

---

* Check labels. Many brands have switched to a combination of saccharin plus aspartame (NutraSweet), a sweetener composed of two proteins that may be no safer than saccharin.

† Cocaine is an alkaloid, like caffeine, but it is extracted from the leaves of the *Erythroxylon coca* plant and other species. Like coffee-bean derivatives, it causes the blood vessels to constrict in the brain because it stimulates the entire central nervous system. [*Stedman's Medical Dictionary* (Baltimore: Williams & Wilkins, 1977).]

brain called the locus cerules to overreact, resulting in the anxiety and panic often seen in abusers, as found by researchers at Yale's Neuro-Behavioral Laboratory.[24]

For openers, soda is our number-one junk food, now that it has surpassed coffee as our national drink (in 1981, sales of soda exceeded coffee sales by 15%).[25] According to the U.S. Department of Agriculture, the official definition of a junk food is a food with "minimum nutritional value.... A 100-calorie portion of junk food contains less than 5 percent of the recommended daily allowance of any one of the eight basic nutrients."

Cola's got plenty of nothing, except calories. And in the case of diet soda, it's got the carcinogen saccharin as well.

Carbonated soft drinks, especially Coca-Cola, are number three on the Center for Science in the Public Interest's list of America's ten worst junk-food offenders. (Tied for first place are ice cream, because of its fat, sugar, and additives, and Kool-Aid, because of its artificial colors, preservatives, and sugar. Coffee with sugar is in second place.)[26]

Table 9 shows how our favorite typical cola drink compares with our most common fruit juice. Both are sweet and easily available. But almost 40% of our beverage dollar is spent on soda and only 8% on fruit drinks. Why? Because cola contains caffeine and orange juice does not.[27]

But there may yet be another reason to avoid colas even if they are free of caffeine, sugar, and saccharin. That reason is trihalomethane, a chemical that is suspected by researchers at the University of Medicine and Dentistry of New Jersey in Newark of causing cancer. A study by Dr. Mohamed Abdel-Rahman, a university pharmacology professor, found 44 parts per billion of trihalomethane in Coca-Cola, 36 in Pepsi, 27 in Dr. Pepper, and 25 in Tab.

Clean drinks appeared the clear winners—7-Up contained only 3 units of trihalomethane, while Sprite had 7.

Officials from the Environmental Protection Agency consider 100 parts per billion to be a safe level. But it's possible that exposure to trace carcinogens from many sources could produce a multiple effect, say experts.[28]

Caffeine and Kids: The Dangers

Kids love cola. And they're cola's biggest customers. And that's not good.

Children, say many prominent researchers, are more susceptible to excitation (by caffeine) than adults. Doctors at the National Institute of Mental Health recently fed a moderately large amount of caffeine (equivalent of two cups of strong coffee) to a group of boys between the ages of 8 and 13 who normally consumed little caffeine. The result? The boys experienced restlessness, nervousness, nausea, and insomnia. Their learning ability was mildly affected as well.

Questions about caffeine and kids were first raised by an FDA advisory group in 1978. A study by Dr. Judith Rapoport at the National Institute of Mental Health indicated that children consuming six cans of cola a day, or its equivalent in other forms (a total of about 300 milligrams), showed symptoms of hyperactivity. Other studies have been equally dramatic.

The universal diet of children with behavior and learning problems is a diet highest in carbohydrate food, in sweets, and in foods prepared with sugar, such as soft drinks. They not only affect the behavior of children, but damage teeth and arteries. "Children are also highly susceptible to the effects of caffeine, which excites the central nervous system, and so caffeinated soft drinks may play a role in school behavior problems," says the Feingold Association of Washington, D.C., adding that "junk foods are responsible for fully 40 percent of hyperkinetic children."

The amount of caffeine used for medical purposes in many pharmaceuticals is 200 milligrams. Therefore, a 12-ounce cola drink is about one-fifth of a stimulating dose. "A quart of cola contains about 300 mg. of caffeine . . . the toxic dose (for a child) is 500 mg.," according to Dr. Hugh Powers, a Dallas pediatrician.[29]

One can of Mountain Dew or Mello Yello contains as much caffeine as a cup of full-strength adult tea and almost as much as a cup of instant coffee (51 and 52%). In addition, more than 50% of the 8 billion gallons of soda kids guzzle annually contains caffeine.

Bearing in mind that among the caffeine side effects experienced by adults are nervousness, insomnia, heartstroke disorders, gastrointestinal disorders, and even cancer, caffeine's effect on a child is even greater and graver.

According to Dr. Candace Pert, an expert on psychoactive drugs at the National Institute of Mental Health, caffeine profoundly affects children. Behavior changes drastically. Caffeine, she says, may so change a child's brain that his future development is affected.

Another problem, notes allergist Doris J. Rapp, is that cola frequently triggers asthma in children.[30]

At the very least, it causes a lot of pain. "Every holistic center in the country has demonstrated that more than 90 percent of all teenage headaches will disappear within two weeks if [teens] totally eliminate caffeine and refined carbohydrates from their diet. At our center, this percentage approaches 97 percent," says Dr. Walt Stoll of Lexington, Kentucky.[31]

High consumption can cause an imbalance in the body that leads to what specialists call "marginal malnutrition," especially when accompanied by other junk foods, such as chocolate, rich in caffeine and sugar.

"[Colas] are being taken by a number of children and adolescents in absolutely fantastic amounts. I think the record I've seen was 98 gallons of cola in two months," says Dr. Derrick Lonsdale, a nutrition researcher at Ohio's Cleveland Clinic.

Colas could also be setting your child up for an ulcer. Caffeine stimulates the production of both the digestive enzyme pepsin and hydrochloric acid in your stomach. You don't have to drink too much coffee to suffer the payoff— an ulcer.

A recent University of California study of 25,000 caffeine users indicated that cola users had a 50% higher rate of peptic ulcer than noncola drinkers.[32] And according to *The Allergy Encyclopedia*, "Irritation of the stomach or intestine is the most common side effect of methylxanthines [caffeine]. It can lead to nausea and abdominal cramping ... because they stimulate secretion of stomach acid. Patients with ulcers of the stomach should be cautious about using them."[33]

In another study, Dr. Daniel M. Thompson of Wichita, Kansas, reported many cases of hematuria, a condition in which the urine contains blood or red blood cells, which is associated with large consumption of soda pop. He concluded that the soda-pop-drinking habit should be included in the medical questions asked patients.[34]

Worse than giving caffeine to a child is giving it to a baby. Yet we do that, too.

There is at least one study that showed that almost one-fifth of all infants under the age of 24 months were consuming some caffeine, while some 6- to 11-month-old infants were taking in almost 80 milligrams a day. This is equivalent to more than one and a half cans of cola, which, in turn, is almost one-fourth of a drug dose for an adult.

We even feed caffeine to our newborns—that's what a breast-feeding, cola-drinking mother is doing. One report tells of a mother whose infant slept the night for the first time only after the mother kicked her caffeine habit.[35]

And remember, caffeine is a drug that crosses the placenta and affects the fetus. If you are pregnant, even a small amount of cola may be hazardous to your unborn child.

Caffeinated colas, like regular tea, also contain some phosphates, phytates, and tannin, all of which interfere with iron absorption.[36] Phosphates are added as acidifiers to soft drinks to keep the drink bubbly and fizzy.

But according to Dr. Diana Philbrick, Ph.D., of the Department of Physiology of Canada's University of Western Ontario and Dr. Peter Haase of the Department of Anatomy, large amounts of phosphates in the diet of laboratory animals produce the rapid formation of kidney stones. Phosphates also cause bone changes by decreasing calcium levels.[37]

Recommendations

1. Switch to a soda pop such as 7-Up or Sprite, which is free of caffeine and other unhealthy substances, such as trihalomethane (p. 86–87) and tannin (p. 64). Most ginger ales, club sodas, tonic waters, seltzers, root beers, and most fruit-flavored drinks are caffeine-free, too. (If caffeine is added, it must be listed on the label. Pepper beverages, like colas, commonly contain caffeine.)

2. If you must have Coca-Cola, its diet brand, as well as

Diet Pepsi, spare you caffeine but provide saccharin. Unless you can stop after one, settle for natural sparkling water or fruit juice.

3. Discuss your child's dependency on cola with your doctor. It could prevent the development of a serious health problem. Caffeinated cola drinks' worst effects are on children.

4. Do not drink colas if you are pregnant or breast feeding. The smaller the child is, the greater the danger. Colas are habituating, so don't make a habit of keeping them in the house. Substitute a variety of alternatives—fruit juices, herbal teas, and just plain water.

5. Don't use soda to wash down medications. According to Professor Edward S. Brady, associate dean of the University of Southern California School of Pharmacy in Los Angeles, soft drinks destroy the effectiveness of antibiotics, such as erythromycin, penicillin, and ampicillin, because of their acidity. The same is true for antihistamines and narcotic pain relievers like codeine.[38]

6. Remind yourself and your family how financially rewarding it is *not* to drink colas. Drop one fifty-cent can of cola a day from your diet, and in 2 months you'll be $30 richer. (Nutritionally, you benefit by saving on the calories found in over 3,500 teaspoons of sugar.) Plan to buy something as a reward for going without.

7. See recipe substitutes in Chapter 10.

NOTE: The following charts do not list all the available national brands or types of products. And, of course, regional brands are excluded. Remember that formulations change. Read labels, consult your pharmacist, or write the manufacturer if you have questions.

Table 7. Saccharin and Caffeine Content in Diet Colas

Product	Mg. saccharin	Mg. caffeine
Diet Coke	NA*	45.
Tab	99.6	44.4
Sugar Free Dr. Pepper	103.68	42.96
Diet Pepsi	125.52	36.0
Pepsi Light	105.48	36.0
Diet Rite Cola	144.0	36.0

* NA—not available

Table 8. Saccharin and Caffeine Content of Noncola Diet Sodas

Product	Saccharin (mg.)	Caffeine (mg.)
Fresca	73.2	0
Sugar Free Sprite	85.2	0
Diet 7-Up	77.76	0
Diet Ginger Ale (Schweppes)	51.0	0

Table 9. Nutritional Value of Cola and Orange Juice

Drink	Calories	Fiber (mg.)	Calcium (mg.)	Carbo-hydrates	Iron (mg.)	Vitamin C (mg.)	Vitamin A (I.U.)	Potassium (mg.)
Cola (8 oz.)	80	—	—	10 g. refined sugar	—	—	—	—
Orange juice (8 oz.)	90	0.1	0.8	2.4 g. natural sugar	30	100	400	400

SOURCE: U.S. Department of Agriculture No. 8 Handbook.

Table 10. Caffeine Content of Soft Drinks

Product*	Mg. per 12-oz. serving†
Regular	
Mountain Dew	52
Mello Yello	51
Shasta Cola	42
Dr. Pepper	38
Pepsi-Cola	37
Royal Crown Cola	36
Mr. Pibb	34
Coca-Cola	33
Cragmont Cola§	Trace
Health Valley Kola Nut Cola	Trace
7-Up	0
Sprite	0
RC100	0
Patio Orange	0
Fanta Orange	0
Fresca	0
Hires Root Beer	0
Diet	
Diet Mr. Pibb	52
Diet Coke	45
Tab	44
Diet Dr. Pepper	37
Diet Pepsi	34
Diet Rite Cola	34
Pepsi Light	34
Diet RC Cola	33
Diet 7-Up	0
Diet Sunkist Orange	0

SOURCES: Figures are provided by manufacturers and Consumers Union. Formulations are subject to change.

* Regular and diet sodas contain only a "trace" of theobromine and theophylline.

† Content comparison: 6-oz. cup of coffee = 75 to 150 mg. caffeine.

§ Made from decaffeinated kola nut extract, which is 2% caffeine.

Chapter 6

What You Need to Know About Chocolate

Chocolate, says food writer Juliette Elkon, is "America's favorite flavor." It is also a source of caffeine and other methylxanthines.[1]

The cacao bean is approximately 2% theobromine, a central nervous system stimulant very similar to caffeine, which dilates vessels of the brain and heart, expands the bronchi of the lungs, and acts as a diuretic on the kidneys.

What's the difference between chocolate and cocoa? Fat content. Both are processed from the fermented roasted seeds of the cacao tree. Depending on the type of cocoa you buy, the fat content is between 10 and 22%. In chocolate it is roughly twice that.

Chocolate and cocoa also contain trace amounts of the methylxanthine theophylline. The average 2-ounce milk-chocolate bar contains about 12 milligrams of caffeine. A cup of cocoa has twice that amount. That chocolate bar also has 42 milligrams of theobromine. And cocoa has 173 milligrams or more. Coffee has 3 milligrams.

In fact, cocoa contains enough theobromine to bring the total level of addictive chemicals up to that of coffee.[2]

How much do we love chocolate? A whole lot. Last year the per capita consumption of chocolate in the United States was 9.1 pounds, and $3.4 billion was spent on chocolate products of all kinds. Although Americans lag behind Austrians, Belgians, Norwegians, Germans, and the Swiss, U.S. consumption of deluxe chocolates, especially—selling for up to $30 per pound—is growing fast.

And there's no end in sight. Exports of Swiss chocolate rose 27% last year, and according to a recent United Nations report, the world chocolate industry will be up at an annual rate of 6% until 1985, including a 21% growth in developing countries. Last year, American chocoholics even made a best-seller out of a humorous book about our favorite sweet entitled *Chocolate: The Consuming Passion,* written and illustrated by ex-greeting card artist Sandra Boynton.

Our annual consumption of chocolate éclairs alone adds 6 trillion calories to the national diet. Some of us are so addicted we eat chocolate chili and smoke chocolate-flavored tobacco.[3]

Chocolate produces a craving like nothing else. A bimonthly newspaper (with 15,000 subscribers), *The Chocolate News,* printed on brown chocolate-scented paper, publishes news of the chocolate world. "An annual Chocolate Binge Weekend at Mohonk Mountain House in New Paltz, N.Y.," and an article about a nine-day "Chocolate Lover's Tour of Switzerland" that you can take for $1,600.[4]

To explain chocolate's mysterious hold one must look to its subtle chemistry, say researchers. Like coffee, chocolate is a complex substance of more than 300 identified compounds, which explains why no one has ever come close to synthesizing it. (This sets it apart from a relatively simple flavor like vanilla, for which vanillin is considered an adequate substitute.)

Chocolate is kid stuff historically, culturally, gastronomically, even literarily. ("Chocolate" is a corruption of the Nahuatl word *chocolatl,* a combination of the Aztec root for chocolate and the word for water.) Nevertheless, chocolate's wholesome reputation has fallen on hard times.

Chocolate Nutritional and Food Value

Compared to coffee, which may have up to twenty times more caffeine, chocolate and cocoa don't look so culpable. On the plus side, the cacao bean is about 90% digestible and comprises 40% carbohydrates, 23% fat, and 18% protein, with traces of vitamin B-6 (riboflavin) and the minerals calcium and iron. It is chocolate's high content of added sugar that causes tooth decay and obesity. One ounce of milk chocolate provides over 150 calories. And semisweet or dark chocolate actually contains *more* sugar in order to counteract the natural bitterness.

Chocolate is also rich in vitamin A, the anticancer, better-sight vitamin. And the magnesium content of chocolate may be the reason women binge on chocolate to relieve the blues associated with menstruation—magnesium hits a monthly low during the menstrual cycle.

Similarly, a craving for hot cocoa may indicate that the body is low in phosphorus, something that cocoa provides (but then so do other foods that are totally caffeine-free and sugar-free, such as lecithin, soybeans, eggs, and fish).

Chocolate also contains phenylethylalamine, a natural chemical that is unrelated to caffeine or other xanthines and that elevates moods and reputedly puts one in the "mood for love." According to the manager of the nutritional sciences division at Hershey Foods Corporation, chocolate is a coping aid, a reward, a symbol of love and affection.[5]

On the minus side, cacao-bean products all contain caffeine, and, if the product is cocoa, it may contain a lot. South American cocoa, for example, has seven times the caffeine content (42 milligrams) of African cocoa (6 milligrams) per 5-ounce prepared serving.[6]

Chocolate also contains between 232 and 272 milligrams of caffeine's cousin, the xanthine theobromine, while tea contains only 2 to 3 milligrams, and coffee, only a trace. That may be a lot, especially for a small child. A couple of chocolate brownies, two cups of a cocoa drink, and a candy bar and/or two tablets of a caffeine-containing medication* can add up to more than 250 milligrams of methylxanthine—a level considered unsafe for children.

Chocolate is also a major factor in migraine headaches. And because of the oxalates it contains, caffeine can bind calcium in the body, thus leading to the development of ulcers, calcium deficiency, and other maladies. With its 23% fat content and 150 calories per ounce, chocolate makes a heavyweight problem.

BHT, a questionable preservative, is added to most chocolate to prevent rancidity. Even worse, chocolate can turn you into a criminal, a headline in the June 2, 1977, *Wall Street Journal* announced. The report by a North Nassau Mental Health Center psychiatrist concluded that violent behavior is often traced to foods such as chocolate, because it is a highly potent allergen. According to Dr. Jose Yaryura-Tobias, a patient arrested for assaulting and injuring his wife admitted during examination to cravings for chocolate, cola drinks, and coffee, all of which made him

* See Tables 12–15.

calmer for a few hours after use. Dr. Yaryura-Tobias placed the man on a diet low in carbohydrates and high in proteins and vitamin B-6. "He improved within eight weeks."

"While a person who is allergic to pollen suffers a stuffy nose, a person allergic to chocolate . . . may pass out bloody noses," said the doctor.

The History of Chocolate

Chocolate does grow on trees. The *Theobroma cacao* is a short tree, rarely higher than 25 feet. It produces clusters of small flowers that grow directly from its main branches and trunk. The clusters of flowers turn into single fruits in the form of a purplish yellow pod, 7 to 10 inches long and 3 to 4½ inches in diameter, with a hard rind marked by 10 elevated longitudinal ribs. Inside the pod are five cells, each containing five to twelve seeds embedded in soft light-pink acid pulp.

Chocolate is made by roasting cacao beans, pressing them to extract the kernel, and then grinding the kernel, which releases the oil and liquifies it. The cooled viscous liquor, without the addition of sugar, is called the mass. The first machine-made chocolate was produced in Paris, as was the use of chocolate in pastry-making and confectionery. Casparus van Houten in Holland is credited with extracting the butter from the mass, resulting in the dry cake that is ground into cocoa. Two Swiss, Daniel Peter and Henri Nestlé, invented milk chocolate—sugar plus whole-milk solids added to the mass.

The finest confectioners' chocolate, known here as *couverture,* is the bitter mass—a minimum amount of sugar plus additional cocoa butter, mixed for up to 96 hours in machines. Thus, the quality of *couverture* is dependent on the raw product—the roasting, pressing, and mixing. It has a minimum of 34% cocoa butter, although the finest chocolate makers demand even higher proportions. These days, Swiss chocolate, mostly milk chocolate, is industrialized, with only a handful of exceptions. The finest chocolate starts with the beans, and the best ones come from South America, primarily Ecuador. Very good chocolate costs 40% more than lesser quality.[7]

And chocolate has played its part in history. Like corn and turkey, cocoa and chocolate originated with the Aztecs.

Chocolate actually started out as a cold, sugar-free drink made by 16th-century Mexican Indians. The Indians valued chocolate as a special-occasion drink reserved for the gods and royalty. When Hernán Cortés (Hernando Cortez) brought a Spanish force to conquer Mexico in 1519, the Indians offered the conquerors their precious cacao beans as a gift, hoping to save their empire.

The Spanish added sugar and hot water to the bitter brew, and quickly fell under chocolate's sweet spell. Somehow, they managed to keep their new discovery a secret for nearly a century.

But by the early 18th century, the fashion for drinking hot chocolate, or *chachaletto,* was the rage in coffeehouses in Europe and in Colonial America, where it soon outsold both coffee and tea.

Chocolate completed its circle from Europe all the way back to America in 1765, when the first chocolate-processing house opened in Dorchester, Massachusetts.

For 300 years following its discovery by the Spanish, chocolate was served as a drink. Solid "eating" chocolate—formed by combining cocoa butter with the chocolate liquor and sugar—was developed by a British firm in 1847. And "milk" chocolate was developed in 1876 by the Swiss, who added dried milk to chocolate.

Today, the Ivory Coast in West Africa is the leading exporter of cacao beans. And Pennsylvania—home of the Hershey Chocolate Company and M&M / Mars—is America's biggest chocolate-processing state.

Cacao Bean: Health Hazards

Is the 3 ounces of chocolate we eat a week hazardous to our health?

Of the three methylxanthines found in our favorite caffeinated pick-me-up drinks—coffee, tea, and cocoa* or hot chocolate—the one found in the largest amounts in chocolate and cocoa, theobromine, is the least damaging to health. It has no significant effect on the central nervous system.[8]

But it does affect other major organs. And for some of us, consequences may be serious.

Just as the caffeine in coffee and tea may lead to ulcers, so the oxalates in chocolate may lead to kidney stones. And heavy chocolate eaters get big doses of this insoluble compound, which is suspected as the cause of almost 75% of human kidney stones diagnosed in Europe and America. How much of these oxalates do you get in chocolate? Oxalates occur in apples, for instance, at levels of 1.5 milligrams (per 100 grams of apple). It is found in equivalent amounts of cocoa at levels of 623 milligrams.[9]

The oxalates in chocolate also block the absorption of calcium. So chocolate milk not only delivers caffeine, it depletes an important growth mineral.[10]

* Actually, a recent nationwide survey indicated that 86% of the population *never* drinks cocoa.

101

Chocolate is also the most common food with which people associate migraine attacks. In any survey, over 60% of migraine sufferers will probably mention this as a trigger factor. Chocolate has a complicated chemical structure and contains many different amines. According to one researcher, migraine attacks can easily be triggered in many sufferers by administering just one of chocolate's amines.[11]

Chocolate is also a common cause of bed-wetting and abdominal pain, two problems common with use of any food containing stimulants.[12]

Studies indicate that all three methylxanthines found in chocolate products appear to be factors in fibrocystic breast disease. (Women with fibrocystic disease, says Dr. John P. Minton, are four times as likely to develop breast cancer as healthy women.) Of his patients who eliminated all caffeine sources, including chocolate, thirteen out of twenty were disease-free within two months to one year.[13]

Although the level of stimulation is low, compared to coffee, chocolate may have a powerful effect on your child's behavior if he or she is sensitive to chocolate. "Chocolate allergy is a major health problem in the U.S.," says clinical ecologist Dr. Marshall Mandell, director of the New England Foundation for Clinical Ecology.

"An allergic reaction to chocolate can affect the brain by slowing down brain function, making the victim chronically fatigued, drowsy and sluggish. . . . It can also stimulate the brain, creating a drug-like high that makes a person unable to concentrate, . . ." says Dr. Joseph Miller, an allergist at the University of Alabama School of Medicine in Birmingham.

"A large number of people with allergies are bothered by chocolate," says Kenneth E. Moyer, a professor at Carnegie-Mellon University in Pittsburgh. "Food allergies can

102

directly affect the body's nervous system and cause a non-inflammatory swelling of particular parts of the brain which can trigger aggression. . . . Symptoms may vary from feeling angry, irritable or upset, to throwing a temper tantrum and destroying things."[14]

Recommendations

1. You don't have to desert dessert. Carob powder makes a nutritionally superior 100% caffeine-free cocoa *and* chocolate. It is naturally sweet, and every health food store and many supermarkets sell it. It has only one-fifth the fat and fewer calories than chocolate, and the absorption of the calcium in a cup of carob milk is not blocked by oxalates, as it is with chocolate milk.

2. Reduce your use of chocolate and cocoa products. Limit yourself to a small amount each week, or reserve it for special occasions. Restrict chocolate in your child's diet as much as possible, especially if any food allergies or health problems exist. If your diet is deficient in calcium, the oxalates in chocolate can cause a serious nutritional deficiency. Drink milk and take a calcium supplement.

NOTE: The following table does not list all available national brands or types of products. And, of course, regional brands are excluded. Remember that formulations change. Read labels, consult your pharmacist, or write the manufacturer if you have questions.

Table 11. Caffeine Content of Chocolate and Carob

Product	Amount	Mg. Caffeine
Cocoa (prepared)	5 oz.	10-17*
Cocoa (dry)	1 oz.	50
Chocolate syrup	2 tbs.	10-17
Chocolate milk (mixed as directed)	6 oz.	10
Chocolate drink mixes	per serving	1-20 (10 mg. average)
Bittersweet chocolate and baking chocolate	1 oz.	20-35
Milk chocolate	1 oz.	3-6
Carob powder (chocolate substitute)	1 oz.	0

SOURCES: *Consumer Reports,* October 1981. Hershey Corporation, 1982 Bulletin. Chocolate Manufacturers Association. *Tea and Coffee Trade Journal,* January 1978. General Nutrition Corporation, Fargo, North Dakota 58107.

NOTE: Although chocolate in any form, including cocoa, contains modest amounts of caffeine, labels are not required to tell you so because it occurs naturally. When caffeine is an addition, as it is in cola drinks and drugs, it must be noted on the ingredients panel.

White chocolate does not contain caffeine. It is a by-product of chocolate, made from the caffeine-containing cacao bean. The bean is processed into two products: a thick syrup (which manufacturers call chocolate liquor) and cocoa butter. The caffeine stays in the syrup, which is further processed into chocolate itself. And the caffeine-free cocoa butter becomes the main ingredient in white chocolate, along with sugar, milk, and flavorings.

* Five ounces of prepared cocoa also contains 232 to 272 mg. of the caffeine-related stimulant theobromine (according to the Center for Science in the Public Interest, the figure is only 178 mg.). While there are 40 to 60 mg. of theobromine per ounce in almond milk chocolate bars, brownies, chocolate candy, and sweet chocolate sauce, and 30 mg. per ounce in chocolate-flavored cake, rolled sponge cake, cookies, chiffon pie, parfait, doughnuts, candy bars, and peanut butter chips, figures are not available for other foods.

Cocoa and chocolate foods contain only traces (defined as less than 1 mg. per serving) of the caffeine-related xanthine theophylline. Carob powder contains traces as well, according to a 1977 laboratory analysis by Wisconsin Alumni Research Foundation in Madison.

Chapter 7

What You Need to Know About Over-the-Counter Drugs

Even if you don't drink coffee, tea, or cola, that doesn't mean you never touch the stuff. Caffeine is hidden in a large number of commonly used prescription and nonprescription drugs—in doses ranging from 15 to 200 milligrams of caffeine per tablet.

If you take one over-the-counter diet pill—such as Ayds appetite suppressant—twice a day, plus two Excedrins at lunch and two No-Doz at night, and have two cups of percolated coffee, plus one Tab during the day, you've consumed almost 1,000 milligrams of caffeine, five times the therapeutic dose, the level at which adverse toxic effects occur.[1]

Caffeine is often incorporated into cold and allergy remedies to counteract the sleep-inducing effects of antihistamines, and in asthma drugs to relax the bronchial muscles. It is also included in many headache remedies to constrict blood vessels in the head, since dilated blood vessels contribute to migraine-type headaches; in "super aspirins," such as APC, caffeine is combined with aspirin and the painkiller phenacetin* because the combination has proven analgesic properties.

Caffeine appears in menstrual pain-relief products, in arthritis pain relievers, in diuretics, and in stimulants, such as the popular nonprescription drug No-Doz. There are even 32 milligrams of caffeine in a capful of Bromo-Seltzer.

The caffeine in such pills has a potential for greater danger than the caffeine in food and drink. The American Council on Science and Health has reported that caffeine "is not a threat to the health of most Americans. However, some people who consume large amounts of products that contain caffeine may experience health problems, including chronic headaches, sleep disturbances, rapid heartbeat, anxiety and stomach upset."[2]

Drug researcher Edward M. Brecher remarks in *Licit and Illicit Drugs* that "the ordinary coffee drinker ... is rarely tempted to drink seven cups, much less a hundred cups, at a sitting," but pills are easy to abuse.[3]

Brecher states that "many Americans use caffeine in this [tablet] concentrated form. How many, and how much of it they take at a time, is unknown—but ten tablets [of No-Doz] contain a gram of caffeine, enough to produce the symptoms of acute toxicity." He then relates a case reported in the *New England Journal of Medicine* in 1936 in which a patient began taking a grain and a half of caffeine citrate (equivalent to 45 milligrams of pure caffeine) three times a day on the advice of a medical professional, to overcome fatigue and exhaustion, which was interfering

---

* The FDA announced in the fall of 1982 that it will ban the painkiller phenacetin in prescription and nonprescription drugs. Phenacetin causes kidney and blood disorders, and possibly kidney and bladder cancer, if taken in large doses and/or over long periods of time.

with her working efficiency. She also was given phenobarbital for her insomnia. After a year of such dosing, the woman took several of the grain-and-a-half caffeine-citrate tablets, and shortly afterward became silly, elated, and euphoric. As hours passed, she consumed more and more of the tablets, until before a party started she had taken the contents of the box—the equivalent of 1,800 milligrams of pure caffeine. She became confused, disoriented, excited, restless, and violent, shouted and screamed and began to throw things. She also became exceedingly profane. Finally, she collapsed, was removed to a general hospital, and diagnosed as psychotic. Not until the woman was taken off coffee, tea, and caffeine tablets, did she return to normal.

Caffeinism caused by the caffeine in drugs can lead to manic depression, says Dr. William Philpott, director of the Philpott Medical Center in Oklahoma City, who has treated many such cases.

Dr. Philpott relates the case of a patient of his who was agitated, depressed, couldn't sleep, and was breathing heavily and who suffered chronic hyperventilation and had attempted suicide by taking a massive dose of arthritis-strength Anacin. Even though he had been treated with tranquilizers and psychoanalysis, he was using eight or more Anacin pills a day for arthritis, which gave him 250 milligrams or more of caffeine per day. After dropping all sources of caffeine from his diet, "the agitation, insomnia, depression, and hyperventilation all disappeared."[4]

"Ten grams of caffeine . . . the amount of caffeine in forty cups of coffee can cause grand mal seizures, respiratory failure . . . even death," says Philpott.[5] This effect can be achieved with even less caffeine if it is being taken with one or more prescribed medications, as was the case here.

Two ingredients in diet pills are a special peril (see

section "Coffee and Weight Loss" in Chapter 2). "Phenyl-propanolamine, or PPA [sometimes identified as an amphetamine], is minimally effective as a diet aid (appetite depressant) and potentially dangerous because it can stimulate the brain and cause large increases in blood pressure. It can trigger life-threatening damage to the blood vessels in the brain. And in laboratory animals, it has even caused strokes."[6]

The annual retail sales of an estimated 90 percent of the diet-pill market of PPA-based products rose from $80 million in 1978 to between $200 million and $250 million in 1983.

And nobody knows how much riskier PPA becomes in combination with 100 to 200 milligrams of caffeine (see Tables 12–16), since it is in all these medications. Even worse are three-ingredient amphetamine "look-alikes" containing high doses of caffeine, smaller amounts of PPA, and an occasional third drug, such as pseudoephedrine, which the *Annals of Neurology* warns "can severely constrict the veins, causing sudden high blood pressure, headache, and then stroke or seizure."[7]

But even simple aspirin becomes a potentially dangerous addictive drug once caffeine is added to it. For this reason, scientists and doctors in Australia are urging that caffeine be banned from the list of over-the-counter pain-killers.

Although only 5% of the brands of nonprescription pain remedies sold in Australia contain caffeine as an active ingredient, these are the brands most preferred by the majority of those who use such drugs.

As a result, doctors note a large increase in kidney disease caused not by the caffeine in these over-the-counter painkillers, but by the fact that the caffeine in them causes abuse of such analgesics.[8] Caffeine-containing aspirin is not only dangerous, since it gives you two drugs in one, but the government has also categorized it as "of uncertain effectiveness," meaning it's yet another widely used pill that doesn't work.

Using caffeine-bearing beverages to wash down caffeine-containing pills can cause caffeine-induced delirium. Stress researchers Dr. Charles Pierce, Harvard professor of education and psychiatry, and Dr. Michael Popkin, professor of medicine and psychiatry at the University of Minnesota, report that "one man treated downed 400 milligrams of caffeine in the form of two Vivarin tablets two hours after drinking two cups of coffee and three cola drinks. . . . In less than 60 minutes he had developed tremors, impaired memory, altered levels of consciousness, vertigo and sensory disturbances consistent with delirium."[9]

Prescription caffeine tablets are probably the riskiest. Consider Cafergot, a drug prescribed to abort or prevent migraine headaches. Side effects are caused by either the caffeine, the ergot, which is a prescription stimulant considered to be habit-forming, or the combination of the two drugs. Cafergot probably causes far more problems than it relieves. Among the minor and major side effects, according to *The Essential Guide to Prescription Drugs,* are itching, nausea, numbness, tingling in fingers and toes, vomiting, chest pain, decreased or increased heart rate, diarrhea, localized edema, and muscle pain in extremities.[10]

And the same thing is undoubtedly true of similar products, such as Cafermine or Cafertrate.

Recommendations

1. Don't take *any* unnecessary drugs. There are safer nondrug solutions to diuretics, diet pills, and cold remedies. Discuss an improvement in your diet and exercise patterns with a qualified nutritionist or physician.

2. If you *must* take a medication drug, look for brands that are caffeine-free. If you aren't sure, ask your druggist.

3. If you are drinking coffee regularly and taking any drug, discuss with your family doctor the possibility of unhealthy interactions that might result. (See list below.)

Caffeine interacts with the following:

1. *Birth control pills:* may increase blood pressure in susceptible subjects and cause high retention and slower elimination of caffeine.[11]

2. *Diet pills and amphetamines:* may double the adverse stimulant effect of caffeine on the central nervous system.[12]

3. *Lithium:* caffeine in doses over 250 milligrams may change the effect of this medicine.[13]

4. *Cigarettes:* smoking doubles the rate at which the body metabolizes caffeine. (If you're a coffee drinker, this may cause you to drink twice as much.)[14]

5. *Thyroid preparations:* caffeine may increase their effects by raising the body metabolism by approximately 10%.[15]

6. *Sedatives, tranquilizers, and sleep-inducing drugs:* caffeine may decrease their effectiveness.[16]

7. *Monoamine oxidase (MAO) inhibitor drugs:* may cause blood pressure to elevate if taken with caffeine.[17]

8. *Meprobamate (Equanil, Miltown):* may delay elimination of caffeine from the body, causing concentration of caffeine in the brain.[18]

9. *Alcohol:* may counteract caffeine's depressant actions on the nervous system.

10. *Asthma medications (Tedral, Aminophylline, Marax, Theophylline-based medications):* may cause excessive nervousness if taken with caffeine.

There are a number of other interactions:

1. Caffeine causes a loss of water-soluble nutrients, including the B-complex vitamins and vitamin C, through the kidneys and urine.

2. The caffeine in coffee can act as a catalyst between amines you consume (found especially in drugs, foods, tobacco smoke) and the nitrates. These are added to processed meats and occur naturally in spinach, beets, and rhubarb. This may result in the formation of potent carcinogens called nitrosamines.[19]

3. The tannins* in coffee, tea, and chocolate also interact with a wide range of medications, reducing the effectiveness of antihistamines, codeine, pain relievers, tranquilizers, and drugs used to treat ulcers and heart conditions—by as much as 90%.[20]

NOTE: The following tables do not list all the available national brands or types of products. And, of course, regional brands are excluded. Remember that formulations change. Read labels, consult your pharmacist, or write the manufacturer if you have questions.

* See Chapter 4.

Table 12. Caffeine Content of Drugs

Pain Reliever	Mg. caffeine per tablet of capsule
Migralam Capsules	100
Excedrin*	65
Migral (P)	50
Fiorinal (P)	40
Apectol (P)	40
Vanquish	33
Goody's Headache Powder	33
Soma (P) (muscle relaxant)	32
Bromo-Seltzer	32
SK-65 Compound (P) (tranquilizer)	32
APC with codeine (P)	32
Darvon (P)	32
Cope Tablets	32
Empirin Compound	32
Anacin	32
Midol	32

NOTES: P = prescription drug; APC = aspirin, phenacetin, and caffeine.

The *Physicians' Desk Reference* warns that migraine headache preparations, such as Fiorinal and APC with codeine, are "contraindicated for individuals sensitive to aspirin, caffeine or barbiturates."

Phenacetin is an antiinflammatory drug and pain killer due to be removed soon from all medication because of its hazards.

Caffeine figures as of fall 1982. Formulations are subject to change.

This list is not comprehensive.

The FDA has given caffeine a category III E status as a treatment for relief of pain, fever, and inflammation. This means it is considered safe but of uncertain effectiveness.

The amount of caffeine in most aspirin and aspirin substitutes is less than the amount intended to stimulate the circulation and distribute the aspirin more effectively. There is no conclusive proof that it improves the effectiveness of the drug.

* Regular Excedrin contains caffeine, but Excedrin PM does not.

Tylenol and Datril—aspirin substitutes—do not contain aspirin.

Other drugs to reduce pain, fever, or inflammation containing caffeine include Medache, Duradyne, and A.S.A. Compound.

Table 13. Caffeine in Stimulant Drugs

Stimulant	Mg. caffeine per tablet or capsule
Refresh'n	500
Slim-Tabs	200
Vivarin	200
Quick-Pep	150
Tirend	100
No-Doz	100
Caffedrine	90–200
Cafergot* (P)	100
Cafecon	100
Cafermine (P)	100
Cafacetin	100
Enerjets	65

SOURCES: Manufacturers and *New York Times,* March 17, 1983.

NOTES: P = prescription drug; caffeine has a category I rating by the FDA when used as a stimulant, meaning it is considered safe and effective.

Read labels. Some brands are available in more than one form containing more or less caffeine.

The drugs above are commonly used for two purposes: to relieve drowsiness and/or to prevent or relieve vascular migraine-type headaches in their early stages.

* Cafergot also contains another stimulant drug, ergotamine. According to the *Physicians' Desk Reference,* "Ergotamine is an alpha adrenergic blocking agent with a direct stimulating effect on the smooth muscle of peripheral and cranial blood vessels and produces depression of central vasomotor centers. Cafergot is contraindicated in cases of coronary heart disease, kidney or liver disease and pregnancy."

The *Physicians' Desk Reference* also warns that the drug may be habit-forming. It also states, "The toxic effects of an acute overdosage of Cafergot are due primarily to the ergotamine component."

Table 14. Caffeine in Diuretics and Menstrual-Discomfort Drugs

Drug	*Mg. caffeine per tablet or capsule*
Aqua-Ban	100
Aqua-Duce	16.2
Diurex	No amount listed
DTU Petane #1 (P)	16.2
Permathene #2 (P)	200
Midol	32.4
Pre-Mens Forte	100
Odnnil	50
Prolamine	140
Super Ordinex	100
Tri-Aqua	100
Mense	32.4

Table 15. Caffeine in Weight-Loss Drugs

Drug	Mg. caffeine per tablet or capsule
Appedrine	100
Diet Plus	150
Hudson Nu Slim	300
Anorexin	100
Anorexin One-Span	200
Ayds Appetite Suppressant Capsule*	200
Ayds Extra Strength	200
Bio Slim T	140
Dex-A-Diet II	200
Dexatrim	200
Dexatrim Extra Strength	200
Dietac	200
Permathene	140
Prolamine	140

SOURCES: *Physicians' Desk Reference* (Oradell, New Jersey: Medical Economics Company, 1982). *Nutrition Action,* published monthly by Center for Science in the Public Interest. Robert J. Benowicz, *Non-Prescription Drugs and Their Side Effects* (New York: Grosset & Dunlap, 1977). U.S. Department of Health and Human Services, Public Health Service, HHS Publication No. (FDA) 18-1081. *New York Times,* April 21, 1982. James W. Long, *The Essential Guide to Prescription Drugs* (New York: Harper & Row, 1980). Product labels on shelves as of summer 1982.

NOTES: The FDA has assigned no category as yet to caffeine used as a safe or effective treatment for relief of fatigue of premenstrual tension or weight loss.

Menstrual-discomfort relief aids *free* of caffeine include Fluidex, Sunril, and Lydia Pinkham.

See discussion of PPA in this chapter.

* Ayds Appetite Suppressant Candy has no caffeine.

Table 16. Caffeine Content of Cold, Allergy, and Asthma Medications

Medication	Mg. Caffeine
Coryban-D	30
Dristan Decongestant AF*	16.2
Neo-Synephrine Compound*	15
Sinapils	32
Emagrin Forte (P)	32
Cory-y Aid	15
Efed II (P)	125
Phenetron Compound (P)	30
Emprazil (P)	30
CCP (antihistamine)	64.8

NOTE: Many bronchial-asthma relief medications contain theophylline† in amounts ranging from 50 to 250 mg. There are over 50 drugs in this category containing this caffeinelike stimulant, which occurs naturally in tea in amounts of 1 mg. per cup. For example: Accurbron, Azma-Aid Tablets, Constant-T Tablets, Marax Tablets and DF Syrup, Sio-Phyllin 80 Syrup and Capsules, Synophylate-GG Tablets/Syrup, Tedral Expectorant, Tedral-25 Tablets, Theophylline Elixir, Theovent Long-Acting Capsules, Isofil, Theo-Nar, and Cerylin liquid.

* Read labels. Some Dristan and Neo-Synephrine formulations are caffeine-free.

† Theophylline is a xanthine similar to caffeine, according to the *Physicians' Desk Reference*. It possesses actions typical of xanthines: coronary vasodilator, cardiac stimulant, cerebral stimulant, skeletal muscle stimulant, and smooth muscle relaxant. Excessive theophylline doses may be associated with toxicity. Alternative drugs should be chosen whenever possible. "The effect of theophylline can be increased," says *The Allergy Encyclopedia*, "if the patient is a heavy coffee, tea or cola drinker."

Other Miscellaneous Sources of Xanthines

Theobromine, a xanthine found in cocoa, chocolate, and tea, is the principal ingredient in two prescription drugs for cardiac disorders: Athemol and Athermol-N.

Chapter 8

What You Should Know About Caffeine-Related Illnesses

Caffeine—especially coffee drinking—has been implicated in promoting or worsening at least two dozen disorders, from insomnia to cancer. The following presents some of the findings.

Pregnancy, Reproductive, and Birth Disorders

If you're pregnant, you're drinking coffee for two. And if the amount is high—100,000 pregnant women drink five, seven, and even ten to twelve cups of coffee daily in the United States—this may increase your risk of spontaneous abortion or miscarriage. In the United States 2,000 babies are born annually with birth defects. An additional 560,000 conceptions result in stillbirths, miscarriages, or infant death owing to defective fetal development.

Caffeine may play a role in that statistic. How big or how small, we aren't certain.

The results of drinking coffee are just as unpredictable

as coffee itself. Some unpublished studies, according to the March of Dimes Defects Foundation, indicate that caffeine may have been responsible for an increasing incidence of breech deliveries, infants with low birth weight, stillbirths, miscarriages, premature births, and other less severe abnormalities.[1]

Other unpublished studies in the foundation's keeping suggest nothing of the kind.

In 1982 a study cited in the *New England Journal of Medicine* found that low-birth-weight babies and premature deliveries observed by researchers in women who drank four or more cups of coffee a day were really caused by cigarette smoking, not by coffee drinking. In effect, the study reported that coffee was okay if you're pregnant, while cigarettes were not.[2]

In another study, conducted at the University of Washington, in which 1,529 women participated (only six of whom were *not* coffee drinkers), researchers reported to the National Drug Abuse Conference that excessive caffeine may have been responsible for the high incidence of less than normally active infants, as well as newborns with below-normal muscle tone. The same study cited a link between caffeine and miscarriages and fetal deaths during pregnancy.[3]

And a recent Canadian study charting the caffeine consumption of pregnant women aged 26 to 36 found that the expectant mothers in their thirty-eighth and fortieth weeks of pregnancy eliminated 30% less caffeine from their system per hour than nonpregnant adults. Caffeine levels in both mother and fetus were three times higher than in nonpregnant women by the end of pregnancy.[4]

Concern is mounting. If you are pregnant, your doctor, nurse, or druggist may have been one of the 967,000 health professionals to be alerted officially to the dangers of caffeine by the FDA's *Drug Bulletin,* published in November 1980: "FDA advises that as a precautionary measure, pregnant and potentially pregnant women be advised to eliminate or limit their consumption of caffeine-containing products."

If the FDA's message didn't reach you via a health professional, the Center for Science in the Public Interest (CSPI), in a letter to those same health professionals, probably did. "We have carefully reviewed the scientific literature and concluded that the consumption of caffeine increases the risk of birth defects and other reproductive problems. We urge you to consider the evidence that implicates caffeine in reproductive problems. We hope you will counsel your patients who are pregnant to avoid caffeine."

Is a warning that may or may not get to you warning enough? No, says Congressman Andrew Maguire (Democrat of New Jersey), who believes that coffee and tea should bear warning labels to protect developing embryos from the hazards of caffeine. "The government needs to develop a clear and consistent policy on chemicals that cause birth defects as soon as possible, if we are to avoid a tragedy such as Britain, Germany, and other countries experienced with thalidomide,"* he says.[5]

The CSPI believes the link between caffeine and birth defects is serious enough to require the formation of a caffeine/birth-defects clearinghouse. It dramatized these efforts at a Capitol Hill press conference, featuring a Virginia woman whose daughter's birth defects "were almost cer-

---

* Thalidomide, the sedative used especially in Europe in the 1960s, was widely prescribed to pregnant women. Severe birth deformities in babies—including missing or deformed arms and legs—were a side effect.

tainly caused by her mother's heavy coffee consumption during pregnancy." The woman told reporters she had scrupulously avoided alcohol, tobacco, and over-the-counter medications during pregnancy but consumed ten to twelve cups of coffee daily. Her baby was born with missing fingers and toes, abnormalities also seen in several animal studies, including a recently completed FDA test. "The tragedy experienced by this family," said Michael Jacobson, executive director of CSPI, "is one more piece of evidence indicting caffeine as a cause of birth defects."[6]

Other cases have turned up. The CSPI has the records of three mothers who maintained a pregnancy-long habit of twelve cups of coffee a day. All three also bore offspring with missing fingers and toes.* In a recent study of women who had been pregnant, only one of sixteen women who drank a lot of coffee (at least eight cups a day) had an uncomplicated delivery. The other fifteen pregnancies ended in spontaneous abortion, stillbirth, or premature birth.[7]

Does that mean less than five cups a day is a safe number? Nobody knows for sure. Some medical experts believe there *may* be a link between the dosage and the danger. Most doctors agree that what is on the high side for a nonpregnant woman may be *very* risky for a pregnant one.

Some of the studies implicating caffeine have been criticized. Commenting on what he termed "the sheer absurdity of the FDA's thinking," but admitting the danger of excess, Howard Roberts, former director of the FDA's Bureau of Foods, noted that in one experiment, pregnant rats

* Michael Jacobson has asked that all women who drank five or more cups of coffee a day and avoided drugs during pregnancy and gave birth to a child with a birth defect to contact his newly formed Caffeine Clearinghouse to help define the risk posed by caffeine. (Write to Caffeine Clearinghouse, c/o Center for Science in the Public Interest, 1501 16th Street, N.W., Washington, D.C. 20036.)

had tubes inserted into their stomachs and the caffeine equivalent of forty cups of coffee pumped in once a day. "In a 110-pound woman that would equate to an instantaneous consumption of somewhat in excess of 40 cups of coffee, or way in excess of 200 cola drinks," said Howard.

Professor Peter Dews of the Harvard Medical School agrees. "Most pregnant women will take two, three, or four cups of coffee. They shouldn't take 5 or 10 times more than the ordinary amount of anything."[8]

In another survey of medical experts who reviewed 10,000 reports, caffeine got a clean bill of health. "Although there are links between caffeine and birth defects, the studies are based on excessive intakes of caffeine," according to Dr. Dean Fletcher, Ph.D., chairman of the department of human nutrition at Washington State University. "Most of the information I've seen indicates a cup of coffee doesn't hurt anyone. There doesn't seem to be any kind of disease or cancer linked to moderate use of coffee."

"Even a pregnant woman can drink two cups of coffee a day," says Dr. John Todhunter, Ph.D., chairman of the biochemistry program at the Catholic University in Washington, D.C., who headed a review of 10,000 studies and articles on the effects of caffeine conducted in 1981 by the biochemistry departments of Catholic University, Washington State University, and the University of Louisville Medical School. "There is no evidence to support reports it can cause birth defects," he said.[9]

On the other hand, many experts agree that a pregnant woman consuming caffeine in any amount could be taking a chance. In September 1980, for example, the FDA released a long-delayed report on an extensive rat study done by FDA teratologist Thomas F. X. Collins, who found that consumption of amounts of caffeine as low as 6 milligrams per kilogram (equivalent to three cups of coffee for a pregnant woman) caused delayed skeletal development, most noticeably in the rats' ribs. Effects at such a low dosage had not been detected previously. Larger amounts, 80 or more milligrams per kilogram (equivalent to about 40 cups of coffee a day), caused partially or completely missing digits on the rats' paws (ectrodactyly). Collins's study demonstrated that, at least in this strain of rat, there was a threshold dose of caffeine below which ectrodactyly did not occur.[10]

"Although caffeine has yet to be established as a toxic to a human fetus," says the March of Dimes Defects Foundation, "any drug that crosses the placenta (as caffeine does) may be regarded as possibly hazardous, especially during the first three months of pregnancy."

If you are average, this advice is even more important. According to a study being conducted by the Epidemiology United at the Boston University School of Medicine, the average pregnant woman continues to take as many as four drugs during early pregnancy, when the embryo is at greatest risk. Women frequently use the drugs before knowing they are pregnant, but *some* medications, including some of those prescribed by physicians, are knowingly used during pregnancy. Aspirin and Seconal lead the list.

And according to Dr. Kenneth J. Ryan, chairman of the department of obstetrics and gynecology at the Harvard Medical School, a good study of a drug to be used by pregnant women might involve a sample of several hundred pregnant women. But if one wanted to find out if the drug was associated with a specific defect, one would need a study population of many thousands of pregnant women, and even if a drug was associated with the rate defect, you might not find it in this sample.

If you continue to use even moderate amounts of caffeine in food and drink during pregnancy, there may be a risk whose outcome no one can predict.[11]

How Caffeine Causes Fetal Damage

The problem is that an infant is unable to metabolize and excrete caffeine until he is about four months of age, so the drug accumulates in his growing system. This, in turn, can have potentially dangerous effects on the heart and nervous system, according to researchers at McGill University. Another study, conducted by the National Institute of Neurological and Communicative Disorders, has shown that mothers who smoke heavily—a habit common among coffee abusers—are at nearly twice the risk for bearing hyperactive children as nonsmokers.[12]

Caffeine readily crosses the human placenta and enters the fetal circulation. This can be harmful because during prebirth development and for the first several days after birth, the newborn lacks the enzyme or enzymes necessary to "demethylate" caffeine.

In one study of sixteen women with estimated intakes of caffeine of 600 milligrams (the amount in five or six cups of brewed coffee or nine cups of instant) or more daily, there were eight spontaneous abortions and five stillbirths. Two women gave birth to premature infants. Only one heavy coffee drinker had a normal delivery.[13]

In another study, the reproductive rate loss was even higher when the male's daily intake of caffeine was greater than 600 milligrams, as was the daily intake of the mother-to-be. "Altered patterns of reproductive outcome may be male-mediated," concluded researchers.[14] A woman doubles her potential for trouble if her husband has the habit, too.

Meanwhile, a West German study conducted in the fall

of 1982, involving almost 1,000 rats getting huge doses of caffeine in drinking water (the equivalent of 90 cups of coffee ingested by a 160-pound male), showed no increased tumor incidence when compared to control animals. What did occur was depressed weight gain and a cessation of sperm production toward the end of the study.[15]

Caffeine's role as a mutagenic (gene-damaging) agent is not new. In 1948 it was reported that caffeine had caused genetic malfunctions and mutations in some types of bacteria.

By 1950, chromosome damage in both cancer cells and human white blood cells had been observed. Caffeine has also long been suspected as a teratogen (abnormal-growth agent).

According to the March of Dimes Defects Foundation, which has been assessing caffeine hazards with regard to the human fetus, it is possible that the body's cells confuse caffeine with one of the components of DNA (deoxyribonucleic acid), which it resembles. Thus, caffeine is permitted to enter body cells, saturate all the tissues, including the fetal gonads, and disrupt the genetic code.[16]

Another theory is that caffeine is *not* a mutagen in humans, but poses its genetic threat by blocking the process by which DNA is made or repaired—especially after it has already been weakened by previous exposure to chemical threat from radiation, for example.

Other researchers are looking into the possibility that the mutagenic and teratogenic damage caffeine does may be caused by one of its breakdown products—which is not identical for every species.

A fourth possibility is based on the physiological fact that because caffeine lingers almost 40% longer in the body of a pregnant woman, this prolonged exposure to caffeine may be what makes caffeine doubly life-threatening.[17]

Human studies are not yet completed, but there is evidence from the results of animal studies. Hens produced fewer fertile eggs when they were inseminated with the semen of caffeine-treated roosters.

Caffeine gains access to the uterus and the testes, where it affects sperm viability and sperm production, say Paul S. Weathersbee and J. Robert Lodge, of the University of Illinois.[18]

Caffeine isn't the only harmful substance in coffee, tea, and chocolate that poses a threat to the unborn and to the nursing infant. According to Jane E. Brody, "Theobromine can also be transmitted to nursing infants in breast milk, though the amounts are usually insignificant. As much as 2% of the caffeine ingested by the mother is transmitted to her infant. Some nursing mothers report that chocolate upsets the baby's digestive tract."[19]

Coffee and Cancer

Does coffee cause cancer?

Since caffeine upsets the entire nervous system and the normal functioning of all the glands in the body that control all our physical and mental functioning, it is not out of the question.

Coffee has been implicated by several recent studies as a definite cause of cancer of the pancreas, stomach, and bladder. *The Lancet,* a prestigious British medical journal, reported that coffee drinking is definitely responsible for a large percentage (25% in men, and 50% in women) of all bladder-cancer cases.

Combining figures from the National Coffee Association and other major research groups, the average U.S. coffee drinker is consuming coffee at a rate that nearly triples the risk of pancreatic cancer. In fact, 10% of all coffee drinkers who quit say that the "fear of cancer" was their motivation.

Cancer of the Pancreas

Recent studies conducted by the Department of Epidemiology of the Harvard School of Public Health and sponsored by the National Cancer Institute indicate that more than 50% of all pancreatic cancers can be potentially attributed to coffee consumption. Cancer of the pancreas is one of the most common fatal malignant diseases in the United States—ranking fourth after cancer of the lungs, colon-rectum, and breast. Of the 24,000 cases on record in 1981, 22,000—more men than women—were fatal. Pancreatic cancer is 5% more fatal than lung cancer, which killed 86% of its victims in 1981, according to the American Cancer Society.

The pancreas, one of the body's most vital organs, situated just behind the stomach, is an oval seven-inch-long organ that secretes digestive enzymes into the small intestine. These help your body turn food into fuel.

In one study by Harvard University, which involved a total of 1,013 patients in 11 large hospitals in Boston and Rhode Island, data were obtained on the smoking and coffee-drinking habits of 369 diagnosed pancreatic cancer patients and 273 individuals with other types of cancer, as well as 371 patients hospitalized with noncancerous diseases.[20]

The risk of cancer of the pancreas was found to be 2.6 times greater for male coffee drinkers and 2.3 times greater for female coffee drinkers than for noncoffee drinkers.

Women who drank more than three cups of coffee a day showed a three times greater risk of pancreatic cancer than noncoffee drinkers.

The study also showed "a consistent association of pancreatic cancer with coffee drinking within each category of smoking, and the data for all smokers and non-smokers showed a consistent trend with coffee drinking after adjustment for smoking."

In another study with almost 100 subjects—made prior to the Harvard study—researchers found an even higher level of pancreatic cancer among drinkers of decaffeinated coffee.

Not everyone accepts the conclusions reached by this study team.

According to Dr. Alvan Feinstein, Yale professor of medicine, there are fundamental problems in the Harvard investigations. Chief among them is the failure to confirm whether the reported increase in pancreatic cancer in this country really represents *new* cases or just better identification of the malignancy.

Columbia University epidemiologist David Rush questions the methods used to determine coffee's involvement. "There are data on normal coffee-drinking patterns," he points out, "and the controls [used] are aberrant for some reason." He praises the study, but objects to the choice of controls, drawn largely from patients suffering from gastroenterological problems.

Other skeptics have questioned whether women are really different from men in their physiological response to coffee.

While conceding that the studies do not prove conclusively a cause-and-effect relationship, and that much broader testing of larger groups would be necessary to provide indisputable evidence, director of the study Dr. Brian MacMahon, professor of Harvard's Department of Epidemiology (who gave up coffee himself in the course of his investigations), says, "Our data suggest that if no coffee were drunk, the incidence of pancreatic cancer would be halved."

If cancer *doesn't* directly result from drinking coffee, *not* drinking it can improve your chances of a cancer-free life. One proof is the low incidence of cancer of the pancreas and other organs among Mormons and Seventh-Day Adventists. Both religious sects urge their members to abstain from coffee and smoking, and their cancer rate is 75% lower than it is for the rest of us.

What does this mean to you? If you are one of the 75 million Americans who drinks two cups of coffee a day, your risk of developing pancreatic cancer may be 80% higher than for noncoffee drinkers. And the more you consume, the riskier it gets. At five cups a day, you more than triple your risk of pancreatic cancer.[21]

Bladder Cancer

If you are a male smoker exposed to industrial chemicals, your chances of contracting cancer of the urinary tract are high. Regular coffee drinking increases the risk.

In a Canadian population-based study of newly diagnosed bladder-cancer patients, 480 pairs of male and 152 pairs of female patients were interviewed about their use of health-hazardous substances, including smoking, use of nonmunicipal water supplies, exposure to high-risk industrial chemicals, and coffee-drinking habits. A second group of healthy individuals were also studied as a "control" group.

Results? Both coffee consumption and regular use of

cola drinks were linked to an increased risk of bladder cancer. The increased risk among men who drank two to four cups daily was about 1.5 times greater than for regular and instant coffee users. Oddly enough, instant coffee proved more dangerous than regular coffee. And the increased risk of bladder cancer did not appear to be dose-related. The risk difference between two cups and four or more was insignificant.

According to the *Journal of the National Cancer Institute,* other studies have come to similar conclusions.[22]

One reason the studies linking coffee consumption and bladder cancer are not as conclusive as experts would like is that few of them consider coffee alone. Heavy coffee drinkers are often smokers as well. This was a criticism of the investigations conducted in 1971 by Dr. Philip Cole of the Harvard School of Public Health, who uncovered an unusually large number of coffee-drinking females with bladder cancer—considerably higher than among abstainers. Men who drank coffee were at a moderately increased risk over men who did not.[23]

But many of Dr. Cole's subjects were smokers as well as coffee drinkers. And there is an acknowledged increased incidence of bladder cancer among smokers. (Certain soluble chemicals in cigarette smoke are excreted with urine, some of which have proved to be powerfully carcinogenic when administered to animals.)

A second significant study of coffee's possible link to bladder cancer was conducted in 1973 by the cancer authority Dr. Irwin Bross of the Roswell Park Memorial Institute in Buffalo. Bross concluded that coffee drinking was probably of little significance in the development of bladder cancer in women, and only slightly increased the risk of bladder cancer in men.

Among the more recent studies is one released in January 1982, in which the National Cancer Institute concluded that the risk of urinary bladder cancer from coffee drinking is very small—even insignificant.

What is the real risk? Cigarette smoking, say the researchers—which explains why coffee drinkers who also smoke have a higher incidence of bladder cancer.[24]

If coffee is not a carcinogen, it's the next worst thing—a catalyst of the carcinogenic process. In 1973 the *British Cancer Journal* reported a correlation between coffee drinking and cancer of the kidneys. Per capita coffee consumption in the United States is five to six times greater than in Great Britain, yet the studies show that the mortality rate from cancer of the kidneys is just slightly higher in the United States.

Why? "If coffee drinking is a factor in the development of cancer . . . it is not on the basis of what we call a 'dose relationship,' where the more coffee consumed, the greater the risk of cancer. . . . Dose relationships are always important in assessing epidemiological studies—unless, of course, the agent in question (coffee, in this case) acts as a catalyst, not as a cause . . . [and] coffee's role in the development of cancers of the bladder and possibly the stomach and kidney may be just that—catalytic," concludes Dr. Donald R. Germann, co-author of *The Anti-Cancer Diet.*

This means that coffee makes the development of cancer more likely when a heavy intake is combined with other foods containing nitrites, or nitrates and amines.

Nitrates, says Dr. Germann, are harmless substances that occur everywhere. They are found in large amounts in some vegetables, such as rhubarb, spinach, and beets. They preserve color in food, for example, bacon, cured lunch meats, and smoked fish, and prevent spoilage. Unfortunately, when these substances combine readily with compounds called secondary amines in your stomach, nitrosamines may be formed, which Germann describes as "highly potent carcinogens. ... From two to five parts per million of one kind of nitrosamine (dimethylnitrosamine) in the daily diet of rats have resulted in cancer. One-time exposure to larger doses has also produced malignant tumors. Nitrosamines are among the few compounds that appear to cause cancer in all members of the animal kingdom. All animals exposed to them, including monkeys, eventually develop cancer of one kind or another."[25]

Amines are found everywhere—in food, drink, tobacco smoke, and drugs, including tranquilizers (such as Valium), sedatives, and cold remedies. It has been estimated that up to 50% of the drugs in any pharmacy contain amines. They are also manufactured by the body.[26]

In April 1975, B. C. Challis and C. D. Bartlett, organic chemists at the Imperial College in London, published a study of their investigations of the possible carcinogenic effects of coffee consumption. They reported that even when nitrites and amines were diluted in a large volume of liquid, the nitrosamine yield increased tenfold when as little as one-third of a cup of coffee was added to the solution.[27]

How to protect yourself?

1. Avoid drinking coffee with meals containing amines or nitrate-rich foods or drinks. Don't wash down medications (many contain amines) with coffee.

2. Take vitamin C with every meal to prevent the amine-nitrite reaction—or at least with meals where amines, nitrites or nitrates, and coffee may all be present.

Heart Disease

Heart disease and vascular disorders are the number one killers in the United States today. Factors in their onset include diabetes, cigarette smoking, or a heavy-stress occupation. Genetic background also increases the risk of developing chronic degenerative heart disease.

Coffee doesn't help, either. Caffeine has a profound effect on the heart, causing heart palpitations, premature beats, and abnormally fast and slow heartbreats. Coffee, in particular, has been associated with both low and high blood pressure. And both regular or decaffeinated types have been linked to the type of heart disease called myocardial infarction.

In 1972, the Boston Drug Surveillance Program confirmed that five to six cups of coffee a day increased the risk of heart attack by 50 to 100%.[28]

At the same time, it was shown that coffee could alter human glucose-response curves so that drinkers tested out more diabetic after drinking coffee than before.

In one of the earliest studies, 276 myocardial infarction patients from eight hospitals in the United States, Canada, New Zealand, and Israel and over 1,000 control patients with other diseases were used.

In the second, the researchers Hershel Jick and Dennis Slone compared 440 patients from 24 Boston-area hospitals with more than 12,000 patients with other diseases.

The conclusion drawn in both cases was twofold: patients who daily drank one to five cups of coffee, both regular and decaffeinated, ran twice as much risk of developing myocardial infarction as nondrinkers; those who drank six or more cups a day ran a risk that was 110% higher.

Also, Jick and Slone noted that subjects consuming equivalent amounts of caffeine from tea, rather than from coffee, did not run the same risk, while the subjects drinking decaf did, focusing attention on the coffee bean itself rather than the caffeine it contains.

Other researchers point to the "total adult population"

study conducted in Finland, which concluded that heavy coffee drinking was a main factor in the onset of both myocardial infarction and CAD (coronary heart disease) fatalities.[29]

A recurrent criticism of both studies is that the studies were conducted with patients who were already ill. Critics of the Jick-Slone study also point to another, better-known study: the Framingham Heart Disease Epidemiology Study conducted under the sponsorship of the National Institutes of Health. Included in the Framingham study were over 5,000 subjects whose health patterns were charted for 20 years in an attempt to uncover a connection between dietary habits and heart disease. There was none, the report concluded.

Still other critics insist that coffee becomes a causal factor only when it adds insult to injury—when the drinker is also a heavy smoker or an alcohol abuser, for example.[30]

If you already have heart trouble, the danger of coffee may be greater. In a 1973 study of 440 patients with acute myocardial infarction, Jick found that the disease was seen 60 to 120% more frequently in coffee drinkers.[31]

And Professor Ronald J. Prineas of the University of Minnesota School of Public Health says more than nine cups of caffeinated coffee increased the incidence of abnormal heart skips. "For people who have suffered heart attacks, VPB [ventricular premature beats] incidents are an absolute proven serious health risk."

Heartbeat Irregularities

Caffeine is used medicinally and legitimately as a potent lung and heart stimulant, which is why it shouldn't be abused recreationally for the same purpose.

The amount of caffeine in two cups of coffee can cause

life-threatening heart-rhythm changes in some people and can briefly produce change in nearly everyone's heartbeat, concludes a study by Dr. Stephen Schaal, professor of medicine at Ohio State University, of all patients with heart problems and healthy volunteers.

"In every patient that gave us a history of caffeine sensitivity, we could induce sustained disorders by giving them caffeine," Schaal said, "even in people without heart problems and who *aren't* sensitive to caffeine, although caffeine increases blood pressure and the heart rate briefly. Coffee and intravenous injections of caffeine were used experimentally; researchers said drinking tea or caffeine-containing soft drinks could give similar results."[32]

Research has shown that abnormally fast heartbeats (tachycardia), as well as slower than normal heartbeats (bradycardia), extra contractions between heartbeats (extrasystoles), irregular heartbeats (arrhythmias), abnormally low blood pressure (hypotension), and abnormally high blood pressure (hypertension) all occur because of caffeine.

If you want to double your chances of developing what the medical profession calls ventricular premature beats (VPB), cardiac irregularities, or abnormal heart skips, as little as four cups of coffee or nine cups of tea a day should do it, if you keep it up long enough.

If you're over 40 years of age, you should limit your intake, advises Dr. Prineas, who headed a recent study on coffee and tea drinking at the University of Minnesota.

Prineas's study of 7,252 men aged 38 to 57 found that the number of abnormal heart skips increased with the amount of coffee or tea they drank.

The trouble with coffee drinking that results in VPBs is that VPBs are not potentially fatal in themselves. However, they do increase the risk of heart diseases. Skipped beats can cause the already-damaged heart to start beating uncontrollably, for example, and that can lead to death. VPBs can also be dangerous to people who have no known symptoms of heart trouble. Since a large proportion of the population has severe coronary atherosclerosis (clogged arteries)—without experiencing any symptoms of heart disease—they run an increased risk from VPB.[33]

Blood Pressure

Caffeine damages the heart and vascular system, and, in the right amounts in the right individual, it increases the amount of FFA (free fatty acids) in the blood.

In November 1965 it was found that plasma FFA in the body was significantly elevated after the consumption of coffee. This condition signals heart disease. The data suggested that the caffeine in the coffee was responsible for the rise in blood fats. It has been shown that increased plasma FFA predisposes a person to a rise in lipoprotein lipids, which in turn increases the possibility of coronary heart disease.

Also, studies point out that a high level of caffeine in the blood increases the amount of cholesterol circulating in the arteries.[34]

Many physicians advise against drinking more than a cup or two of coffee when the blood pressure is borderline or when the patient is 40-plus, and especially if both conditions prevail. "Caffeine might enlarge the population of 'hypertensive subjects' by increasing the pressure of those with borderline hypertension," concludes a report appearing in the *New England Journal of Medicine*.[35]

But many physicians, according to the cardiologist and

marathon runner Dr. George Sheehan, medical editor of *Runner's World* magazine, believe that "so far, coffee—the drink that wakes you up in the morning—seems to be holding up under standard scientific assaults. . . . Even up to nine cups a day doesn't have any bad effect on blood pressure . . . the conclusion reached in a study of 87,000 IBM Corporation employees. The same incidence of normal, borderline and high blood pressure was found in groups drinking no coffee, 1–3 cups daily, 4–8 and more than nine. (Blood pressure readings were done in semi-basal state. That is, [the subjects] had abstained from food for 12 hours, had not smoked for 30 minutes and had been resting for about 15 minutes before the examination.)"[36]

Another study that gives caffeine a clean bill of health as a factor in cardiovascular disease was conducted by scientists at the Duke University Medical Center. "People who drink five or more cups of coffee a day suffer no greater risk of mortality than those who drink little or none," said the study's directors, who interviewed 2,350 adults over 4½ years in rural Evans County, Georgia, to learn their coffee-consuming habits.

Central Nervous System Disorders

Studies indicate that we all think better and work harder with a little coffee in our systems. Vast quantities of coffee are what kept the nineteenth-century French writer Balzac on the ball for 16 hours at a stretch while writing his celebrated novels. Coffee even helps us move faster.

"[If you] stimulate the sympathetic nervous system by ingesting caffeine 60 minutes before exercise, you observe a 19 percent increase from exercise time to exhaustion . . . using 4–5 milligrams per kilogram of body weight, or roughly two cups of coffee. . . . This application of the most

American of breakfast beverages to running is seemingly revolutionary in nature—and almost as revolutionary in its simplicity. . . . In a more recent study, it was found that the taking of a similar caffeine drink before two hours of exercise produced a seven percent increase in the amount of work that could be performed."[37] Despite the fact that the subjects of the test cited had no idea what they were drinking, in every case they found the exercise markedly easier after the caffeine. The explanation for this enhanced performance following the caffeine is complex, but directly related to a greater burning of fat. Without the use of caffeine, subjects obtained 22% of their energy from fat. After the caffeine drink, fat contributed almost 40% of the total energy demands. "Reliance on fat," continued the researchers, "lessens the use of precious muscle glycogen, thereby delaying the point of exhaustion."

"The nervous system stimulation you get from 200 milligrams of caffeine," according to Richard H. Zander, "is the equivalent of 10 mg. of amphetamine sulfate."*[38]

Coffee introduced into your gastrointestinal tract is easily absorbed by the body. It reaches a peak in the bloodstream after about 60 minutes, then passes rapidly into the central nervous system (CNS).

Caffeine's first target is the cerebral cortex and the medulla. It also stimulates the three systems that are responsible for breathing, blood-vessel dilation, and operation of the vagus nerve, which provides energy for the functioning of the larynx, lungs, heart, esophagus, and most of the abdominal organs.

Adjusting your metabolism has a price. It produces only short-term benefits and long-term ills.

Coffee may improve alertness and thus productivity, for

* More on coffee as an energizer in Chapter 1.

example, but not necessarily the product. According to a recent study at the University of Oklahoma, male and female students were grouped in four caffeine-consuming groups—abstainers and low consumers of coffee were C-plus students, and the moderate and heavy coffee drinkers had C-minus averages. Results were "striking," according to Dr. Kirby Gilliland, who ran the tests, indicating a strong negative relationship between caffeine consumption and success in academic performance. "Heavy caffeine users reported more negative effects from their caffeine intake than did the other groups, including digestive problems such as heartburn and diarrhea."

And there is lots of evidence that caffeine makes you duller. In another survey, high school students in Dallas, Texas, who consumed high levels of both sugar and caffeine daily, also scored the lowest marks.

And if you're allergic to coffee beans—a large percentage of us have hidden coffee allergies—coffee drinking can make a real dummy out of you. Dr. William G. Crook is "convinced that what you eat (and drink) can make you dull, stupid and hyperactive."*[39]

In fact, whereas 10% of us eliminate coffee from our diets because of a risk of cancer, the largest percentage of quitters cite coffee's effects on their minds and nerves as the motivating factors.[40]

The following discusses some of the central nervous system disorders coffee causes.

Glandular Exhaustion

Caffeine in your system is like the preservatives in food—it doesn't improve anything, it just extends shelf life. Caffeine permits you to overextend yourself. How does it do this? According to a research team headed by Dr. Solo-

* More on coffee as an allergen in Chapter 1.

mon Snyder, director of neuroscience at the Johns Hopkins School of Medicine, caffeine inhibits the natural mechanism that tells your body when to slow down. Snyder said the discovery may point the way to improved drugs. His research indicates that caffeine may block the action of a compound called adenosine, one of the building blocks of DNA, involved in cellular energy. Its crucial function seems to be as a "neuromodulator," or nerve depressant. Snyder says that caffeine's chemical cousins—theophylline and theobromine—derive their stimulating properties from their relative's ability to block the functioning of adenosine.[41]

Low Blood Sugar

Coffee makes a major contribution to another disorder affecting both the glands and nerves—low blood sugar, or hypoglycemia, a minor disorder that often leads to major diseases and that is more prevalent in the United States than diabetes, afflicting at least 50% of the population. Fatigue and irritability are the common symptoms, but anything from allergies to schizophrenia is possible.

A rapidly changing blood-sugar level makes you prone to fatigue. "It can scramble your reasoning faculties and roller-coaster your emotions," according to Dr. Samuel Arnold, a clinical assistant professor of urology at Rutgers Medical School. "It's better to delay eating anything at all rather than having just coffee and doughnuts for your breakfast."[42]

When you consume too much caffeine, it stimulates the adrenal cortex, which in turn releases hormones that stimulate the liver. The liver than breaks down some of its glycogen store into glucose. The glucose then pours into the bloodstream and triggers the release of insulin. There is also evidence that indicates that a deficiency of the B-complex vitamins that help in the metabolism of carbohydrates can be a factor in this condition, and caffeine destroys B vitamins. (The use of other drugs, such as antibiotics, hormones, stimulants, anticoagulants, and tranquilizers, has also been cited as a causative factor in low blood sugar.)

One of the most widely accepted diets in the treatment of hypoglycemia is the high protein/low carbohydrate diet. This plan is based on the work of Dr. Seale Harris, who first described the disease and its proper treatment over 50 years ago. No liquor, strong tea, coffee, soda, chocolate, or cola beverages are allowed. It gets results.

Diabetes

Coffee also contributes to high blood sugar, or diabetes. Researchers who studied the uptake of glucose in isolated fat pads of rats observed that caffeine significantly reduced glucose uptake.[43] And in another study, it was reported that coffee lowers glucose tolerance in maturity-onset diabetes.[44]

"Over the years, caffeine has been linked to other diseases such as ... diabetes.... However, to date there is no firm evidence proving that caffeine causes any of these problems though it may aggravate existing problems," according to *The Harvard Medical School Health Letter*.[45]

"What makes caffeine a specific diabetes negative is its tendency to raise the blood sugar. Total elimination of caffeine is advisable if not imperative," advise June Biermann and Barbara Toohey, authors of *The Diabetic's Book*.

Mental and Emotional Illness

Too much caffeine can lead to a form of emotional and mental illness called caffeinism (discussed in Chapter 1), or caffeine intoxication.

Consider the behavioral effects of large doses of caffeine in animal experimentation. Several research teams have reported that rats fed massive doses of caffeine become aggressive and launch physical attacks against other rats. A caffeine-crazed rat may bite and mutilate himself. Automutilation is so acute and intense in some rats that the animals die from hemorrhagic shock.[46]

According to Dr. Kirby Gilliland and Dr. Gordon Deckert, experts on caffeinism, almost a fifth of the country's coffee drinkers may be victims. "We have seen patients treated unsuccessfully for anxiety neurosis for years. Tranquilizers and psychotherapy didn't work for these people.... But when it was discovered that these patients consumed heavy amounts of caffeine a day, and the caffeine was removed from their diets, extreme anxiety just disappeared."[47]

And Dr. Emmanuel Cheraskin, one of the authors of *Psychodietetics,* warns, "Whether you are now experiencing emotional upsets or not, if you are a heavy consumer of coffee (or) cola drinks . . . you had better take some dietary precautions . . . But remember, the everyday addict, who habitually uses caffeine [and] nicotine . . . needs help along with the stereotyped addict hooked on illicit drugs."

Coffee accounts for the depression experienced regularly by one out of every six Americans. One study at the University of Michigan Medical School has found a direct connection between the amount of caffeine consumed and the degree of depression among 83 psychiatric patients. Of the heavy users (seven cups or more), 50% were seriously depressed.

Thus, abuse of caffeine—a nonprescription drug—often leads ironically to abuse of prescription drugs—chiefly tranquilizers and barbiturates—to counteract caffeine's side effects.

141

Many psychiatrists prescribe antipsychotic drugs for their patients. Often patients are already suffering from nutritional deficiencies, and drugs further this malnutrition. Antipsychotic medications may control the condition for which they were prescribed, but they can interfere with nutrient metabolism and cause new mental abnormalities to appear.[48]

Caffeine and Gastrointestinal Distress

Over a third of all coffee drinkers who kick the habit do it because it gives them gastrointestinal trouble* even when consumption is minimal, and often even when it's just decaffeinated.

Statistics indicate that up to 50% of the coffee-drinking population suffers from heartburn, often accompanied by diarrhea, gas, or both. And heartburn can result as easily with two cups as it does after fifteen.

One study examined 57 heartburn-troubled drinkers who had either given up coffee (35%) or reduced their intake (65%). When coffee was reintroduced into each individual's system through nasogastric tubes, 50% suffered from gas—ranging from bloating, belching, and passage of flatus; 39% developed diarrhea; 9% complained of chest pains; and 11% experienced nausea.[49]

As mentioned earlier, it appears that you may not save your stomach from upsets by switching to decaffeinated coffee. In fact, switching to *any* roasted grain beverage may be contraindicated, say researchers, because it's the roasting process itself that releases the oils—the culprit—and acids, which in turn produce gastric irritation.

---

* If you don't believe coffee can be death on your digestive system, watch how a cup of cold brewed java cuts the grime and grease on your barbecue grill.

That burning sensation beneath the breastbone occurs when a spastic backflow of acid stomach contents flows into the esophagus. This backflow can be caused by an increase or a decrease in lower esophageal sphincter pressure. The sphincter is a muscle that can open and close the port between the stomach and the esophagus.

And it isn't just the caffeine that irritates organ tissues and stomach lining, but also the oils and volatile acids in the coffee bean, which are released by roasting and grinding. This explains why switching to a low- or no-caffeine brand may not reverse your gut reactions from bad to good either.

If you are habituated to dark-colored, "full body" brews, there could even be an ulcer in your future. According to the *New England Journal of Medicine,* caffeine aggravates the symptoms of peptic ulcer by stimulating gastric-acid secretion. The component responsible for the acid secretion may be one of the components of coffee other than caffeine. And decaffeinization does not alleviate the problem, because acid secretion is only minimally reduced, continues the report.[50]

In a study by Dr. R. D. Paffenberger of the University of California at Berkeley, which followed the medical history of 25,000 men from their college years to middle age, the coffee-drinking habit was very closely linked to ulcers. Coffee drinkers, says Paffenberger, have a 72% higher chance of developing ulcers than individuals who never use coffee.

If you drink coffee on an empty stomach, you add insult to injury. Coffee's oils disturb the normal acidity of the stomach necessary for digestion, and without protein or fiber from food to buffer this effect, a stressful condition of hyperacidity is made worse by the coffee bean's irritating ingredient.[51]

Adding a protein-rich food before drinking, or putting cream in your coffee, helps. So does avoidance of the dark, oily offenders that include Brazilian roast, Viennese, French, Spanish, and Italian espresso-type coffees.

What's the *good* news? That you *can* get your gastric good health back just by quitting as soon as possible.

While disturbances of the heart, lungs, and central nervous system appear fairly evenly distributed throughout respondent groups regardless of age, gastrointestinal problems appeared more likely to occur among coffee drinkers who had been drinking too much (at least three to eight cups) too long. But this is not always the case. According to Charles Wetherall, author of *Kicking the Coffee Habit,* "Persons who quit [coffee] primarily because it was extremely distressful to their gastrointestinal systems drank little more than anyone else in our survey . . . around eight cups a day . . . [but] some coffee drinkers began complaining about the effects of coffee with as few as one cup per day."[52]

The risks of ulcers and other stomach disorders, in fact, seems to increase in direct proportion to the number of years you spend as a heavy coffee-drinker.[53]

If you're not ready to quit, at least don't couple your coffee with other foods that also upset your stomach. A breakfast meal containing fried eggs, or variations of other fried foods, followed by the use of butter and then coffee is a disaster.

Fibrocystic Breast Disease

If you are a woman between 25 and 50 and using caffeine, the risk is especially great. This population is especially susceptible to a caffeine-linked disorder called fibrocystic breast disease, mammary dysplasia, or fibrous mastopathy, also sometimes called "the breast disease that isn't cancer."

It may not be just coffee. In a recent study of 491 randomly selected undergraduates at a major Midwestern university, 86% of the students were found to use caffeine, mostly through cola beverages. Fifteen percent of the women sampled consumed 500 milligrams or more (equal to about five cups of coffee) a day, and 25% used 250 to 500 milligrams, in contrast to only 3% of the male students who used 250 milligrams or more at any time during the survey.[54]

One out of every six women, or one-fifth of all American women, are afflicted with some form of this benign breast disease. Sufferers are two to eight times more likely than other women to get breast cancer eventually.

It usually affects both breasts, and multiple cysts of many sizes are common. Some cysts may actually grow as large as a hen's egg. They are often painful, especially before menstruation, and sometimes must be surgically removed. And while the cysts themselves are not malignant, a malignant growth may accompany them. Consequently, the disease must be monitored.

What causes fibrocystic disease? It is thought to be a metabolic condition associated with a hormone imbalance occurring in the estrogen-producing years of a woman's life. Fibrocystic disease peaks during the mid- to late thirties. And often all traces of the disease will disappear after menopause occurs.[55]

In many cases, abstinence from caffeine and the other xanthines (this includes chocolate and decaffeinated beverages because they also contain a small amount of caffeine, theobromine, and theophylline) can be both the prevention and the cure. (Nicotine has also been implicated as a causative factor.)

On the presumption that methylxanthine, in the form of caffeine, is the cause of fibrocystic disease, Dr. John P. Minton of Ohio State University eliminated caffeine from the diet of women with symptomatic fibrocystic disease. Of these women, 65% experienced complete clearing of the problem after only 6 months, and only one of the twenty-seven women who did not take Dr. Minton's advice experienced relief. The remaining twenty-six women were required to undergo biopsy to determine if the lumps were cancerous.[56]

In another study by Dr. Minton, which spanned four years and in which 120 women with fibrocystic disease participated, 80 of those who eliminated all sources of methylxanthines from their diets found that their cysts gradually disappeared. They also remained symptom-free as long as they stayed away from all foods, drinks, and medications containing caffeine and related stimulants.* Not only are nodules and pain eliminated by this dietary measure, but the need for surgical biopsies is also eliminated.[57]

Manhattan obstetrician Michael Strongin, like many professionals, is advising his patients to cut back on coffee—to have one cup, two at the most, but better yet, none. About 60% of those who completely give up methylxanthines report less pain and fewer lumps before their menstrual period.[58]

On the other hand, the evidence is not totally conclusive. A study at the University of California that attempted to duplicate Dr. Minton's results didn't come up with the same answers.

* Consult all the tables in the book for substances to avoid.

If you are in your twenties and don't drink much coffee, why should you care? Because a breast-tissue climate conducive to fibrocystic disease is also conducive to breast-cancer cells. Thus, a malignant tumor may grow side by side with a nonmalignant fibrocystic lump. A young woman who now has fibrocystic disease stands a slightly greater chance of developing breast cancer later on in life.

Methylated xanthine intake appears to be linked to prostatic disorders in men as well. Not surprising, since prostate-gland tissue is structurally similar to female breast tissue, this link is unfortunate for men, since fibrous growths on the prostate are more difficult to detect than those in breasts.[59] Both regular and decaffeinated coffees are suspect.

Allergy / Addiction

Is coffee habituating? It must have something going for it, for although the medical profession cites "jitteriness, insomnia and possible damage to overall health" as reasons for cutting out coffee, only 17% of the country's doctors surveyed practice what they preach. And 8% admit to a habit of five or more cups a day.[60]

"So pervasive is the U.S. coffee habit that in some American restaurants the waitress asks if the customer would like a cup of coffee even before she gives him a menu," says food writer James Trager.[61] And why do large numbers of us say yes? Because large numbers of us can't say no. We're addicted.

Addicted, in many cases, is just another way of saying food allergy. An irresistible craving for a food signals allergic addiction.

Allergic food symptoms include everything from head-

147

aches to adrenal exhaustion. And if drinking coffee makes you feel like eating more, even if you just finished eating, blame that on your allergic addiction, too. As one doctor explains, "From chemical receptors in the brain, the adrenal gland receives the message that the blood sugar level is falling, hunger follows and another chemical or nerve impulse dilates the blood vessels in the brain (thus producing headache) in an effort to restore optimum flow of glucose to the brain . . . [and] the body will crave certain foods . . . when they are avoided. . . . Thus the avoidance is actually withdrawal and can produce headaches as well as an intense urge to eat."[62]

This cycle can occur with any food containing caffeine or the related stimulants—chocolate, for instance. "Allergy manifests first as addiction to the very thing that is doing harm. A person at this stage will get a brief pick-up. There is relief of tension and other symptoms, such as headache, on eating or drinking the allergen chocolate or cocoa—and you only feel bad some hours later if another dose of chocolate . . . is not taken . . ." according to Dr. Richard Mackarness.[63] You get into a cycle of pick-up and hangover just like the alcoholic, who is the best example of someone hooked on what, for him, is a self-administered poison in large doses. The symptoms, when you don't get that second chocolate bar or cup of coffee, can be anything from headache to fatigue to serious depression.

For many adults, 300 milligrams, an amount that produces the physical symptoms of hyperactivity in children, is all that's needed to produce dramatic "mood changes," notes Dr. Judith Rapoport in a study she conducted for the National Institute of Mental Health.[64]

Symptoms besides depression are many and varied. Do you get a headache or a pain in your shoulder or leg when you have one or two cups of coffee? Do your ear lobes redden, eyes appear glassy? These are all telltale signs, say allergists. Other allergic responses include mood swings, tension fatigue, and dark circles under the eyes. Either regular or decaffeinated coffee can do it.

If you are allergic to coffee beans, you can add a few unexpected side effects to all of coffee's conventional symptoms. In his book *Dr. Mandell's 5-Day Allergy Relief System,* the Norwalk, Connecticut, clinical ecologist discusses the reactions of a multiple sclerosis victim when tested for sensitivity to coffee extract: "She became slightly nervous and moderately tense, with difficulty in concentrating. Then she felt 'spaced out.' When most patients use this expression it means that things appear to be unreal. It was an effort for her to maintain contact with her surroundings. Next, she had some mild tingling within her lower extremity, which was a familiar symptom to her; it seemed to me that this might be important because it was the leg that she limped with. This coffee test suggested the possibility that some aspect of her MS and limp could be related to the ingestion of coffee."

A "freak" case? Dr. Mandell provides another example: "I started her [the patient] on a diagnostic rotary diet to determine the foods to which she might be allergic. . . . Within minutes after drinking a cup of black coffee, all her symptoms of 'emotional' illness were reproduced in a very convincing manner. . . . She was one of the very few patients I have ever seen where a single factor (coffee) was identified as being the *only* cause of a long-term illness." Management of this case proved to be incredibly simple. "She eliminated coffee, and for the first time in many years, her gastrointestinal tract began to function properly and absorb foods normally. She gained weight after years of being painfully thin."

And if you let your coffee allergy continue? According to

149

clinical ecology specialist Dr. William Philpott, untreated food allergies can lead to the weakening of the entire body. And this, in turn, can cause the onset of a host of degenerative diseases, including arthritis, pancreatitis, heart disease, premature aging, diabetes—and even mental illness.[65]

Other Illnesses

"Most disease today is related directly to the environment. Sickness creeps up on us after long years of breathing bad air, eating false food, smoking, and avoiding recreation. If we accept our current environment at face value, we are almost certain to be tricked eventually into disease, . . ." says Robert Rodale, director of the Soil and Health Society. "Trust that drugs will put you to sleep, wake you up, cheer your days, lessen your worries, and you'll end up a pale imitation of a real human being."

He could have been talking about just coffee and caffeine-related foods. No drug tricks you into disease as readily as caffeine.

One reason is that every cup of coffee depletes vitamins essential for improving health and preventing stress. Coffee is a vitamin antagonist, which means it interferes with the absorption of nutrients from the foods and food supplements we take.

Coffee is also a laxative and a diuretic. It increases urine production, which in turn means loss of water-soluble nutrients, such as the B and C vitamins. It increases loss of minerals such as zinc and potassium, important antistress factors, through the feces.

In a recent study of coffee's effect on thiamine (vitamin B-1), volunteers drank seven cups of coffee in three hours. Eight days later, they drank the same amount of water. On both days, researchers measured the amount of thiamine excreted later in the volunteers' urine. The amount was 45% more on the coffee day than on the water day—evidence, say the researchers, that coffee destroys thiamine because thiamine is a water-soluble vitamin and coffee, a diuretic, flushes such vitamins out of the system. Decaffeinated coffee had the same effect.[66]

And digestive problems created by the irritation of coffee drinking can lead to other nutritional problems, especially a shortage of the fat-soluble vitamins A, D, and E. These are lost—that is, not absorbed—in any disorder associated with digestion: liver problems, gall-bladder problems, pancreatic disorders, such as cystic fibrosis, and any condition that causes chronic diarrhea, something coffee does for many drinkers. Every cell in your body suffers when there is not enough of any given vitamin to perform all the functions for which that vitamin is responsible.

Magnesium deficiency is another possibility. Since all diuretics, and that includes caffeine, also cause excessive loss of this mineral, which is essential for good health. It is an important constituent of both soft tissues and bone, necessary for helping regulate the body temperature, for the working of muscles and nerves, and for the proper manufacture of protein. The richest food sources of magnesium are nuts, soybeans, peas, beans, peanuts, whole-grain cereals, wheat germ, and brown rice.

Minor nutrient shortages can be a factor in many diseases besides the major killers. For example, caffeine may be a factor in osteoporosis, the brittle bone disease that afflicts millions of middle-aged women every year.

In one long-term study of 168 women between the ages of 36 and 45, researchers found that a moderate amount of caffeine (two cups of coffee a day) interfered with absorption of calcium in the diet. A net calcium loss of 22 milligrams per day was recorded. Adding one more cup of coffee resulted in a loss of almost 30 milligrams. A negative calcium balance of only 40 milligrams per day is "quite sufficient to explain the 1 to 1.5 percent loss in skeletal mass per year noted in postmenopausal women," added the researchers.[67]

Coffee is worse news if you're 40 and rheumatic, says Dr. Philip J. Welsh of North Dakota, author of *Freedom From Arthritis*.[68] "Excessive coffee drinking in adults predisposed to rheumatism invites disaster. . . . There is chemical proof to the effect that caffeine is converted into uric acid in the body. . . . Uric acid is one of the many acids, an excess of which leads to trouble."

Coffee drinking can even accelerate the aging process, especially if other stress factors are present in your life. According to Robert Morgan, a psychologist at Wilfrid Laurier University in Waterloo, Ontario, Canada, "Smokers and coffee drinkers tested have shown advanced aging."[69]

Restless legs, a syndrome that occurs independently or in association with night leg cramps, is an extremely uncomfortable, often damaging, continuous movement of the legs. Episodes may last for hours. One recent study suggests that caffeine may be a major factor in producing this syndrome. All fifty-five patients in the study benefited from treatment consisting of avoiding caffeine-containing beverages and medication (often used to counteract the restless-leg problem) and the temporary use of a drug. They continued to benefit only when they kept away from caffeine.[70]

Caffeine may even cause tooth decay. According to Dr. Hal Huggins, writing for the *Natural Foods and Farming Association Magazine*, "Degenerative diseases all come from the same origin, an imbalance in the chemistry of the body. Caffeine causes calcium-phosphorus and blood chemistry to get out of balance.... Phosphorus is the protection of the heart. When phosphorus levels go down, we become more susceptible to dental decay and periodontal disease.... Caffeine comes in about number two after sugar [as an agent that] will make calcium go up and phosphorus go down."

Chapter 9

Sizing Up the Problem:
How Much Caffeine
Is Too Much?

"A lethal dose of caffeine for a healthy adult male," says the *Physicians' Desk Reference,* "is approximately 10 grams, the equivalent of 80 to 100 cups of coffee drunk in rapid succession. But because our bodies can break down caffeine and excrete it rapidly, deaths from overdoses of the stimulant are virtually unknown."[1]

If caffeine is that poisonous, why doesn't it poison us all? Evidence indicates that you just may not be picking up the clues, because cause and effect are sometimes years apart.

As the author of *How To Get Well* puts it, "Caffeine contributes to stress debit ... for which you must pay sooner or later in the form of stress-caused pathological conditions of some sort—like heart disease or nervous exhaustion."[2]

Secondly, everybody has his limits. Like liquor, some of us hold our coffee better than others. That doesn't mean we aren't suffering all the harmful effects. It just means a tolerance has been built up. (See *Coffee as an Allergy*.) In fact, the less affected you feel and the better coffee makes you feel, the more you may have to worry about.

In one study conducted by the Department of Pharmacology at Stanford University, a group of women who were not coffee drinkers were given decaffeinated coffee to drink, and exhibited no unusual symptoms. A second group, consisting of women who were regular five-cups-a-day drinkers, complained of feelings of nervousness and jitteriness, even nausea. When they were given decaffeinated coffee, their irritability increased. But when the researchers gave them regular coffee again, all symptoms disappeared.[3]

Researchers added that "in addition to the effects of caffeine on temper, regular coffee-drinking housewives developed a noticeable drug like dependence on the beverage. . . . When given decaffeinated coffee, the women demonstrated symptoms typical of drug withdrawal in addicts."[4]

Factors such as age, size, sex, and varying states of health account for varying responses to caffeine, too.

Caffeine's effects are unpredictable. Caffeine works as an *anti*stimulant, for example, when used as a medicine to counteract apnea in adults or hyperactivity in children.

But ordinarily it has an undesirable amphetamine-like action, especially since it is usually accompanied by sugar, another stimulant substance found in foods.

And because a child weighs much less than an adult, a can of soda drunk by a child is roughly equivalent to a cup of coffee drunk by an adult, points out Michael Jacobson, director of the Center for Science in the Public Interest, and one cola may produce the caffeine syndrome or "coffee nerves" seen in adults who have had four to five cups of coffee.

155

In other words, physiologically speaking, kids will be kids and grownups will be grownups.

Also, as previously noted, caffeine has a more stimulating effect if you are young and strong. If you are over 60, caffeine may have the opposite effect, and put you to sleep.

What's more, caffeine's side effects, such as acid indigestion, restlessness, insomnia, and headaches, increase as you age, and "tolerance for caffeine often decreases after 60."[5]

Caffeine has an even more deleterious effect if you are unwell in any way. Even a single cup can be way out of line if your mental health is already hanging in the balance, for example. Unstable personalities as measured by psychological personality tests "have anxious reactions to small doses of caffeine. Unstable males in particular become terse and easy to anger."[6]

Also, notes the *FDA Consumer,* combining caffeine with certain foods or medicine can increase caffeine's impact (see pages 110–111), for certain individuals. "The extent of interaction between food and drugs depends on the drug dosage and on the individual's age, size, and specific medical condition . . . [and] the presence of food in the stomach and intestines can influence a drug's effectiveness by slowing down or speeding up the time it takes the medicine to go through the gastrointestinal tract."[7]

One of those affected substances is caffeine. The caffeine in one cup of coffee could have the effect of four, two, or ten cups if taken with drugs. Coffee on an empty stomach is more potent than coffee taken with a meal. Likewise, coffee or caffeine-containing food or drink taken with an oral contraceptive causes more caffeine to be retained and less medication to be absorbed. There is no way of predicting with certainty.

How Much Caffeine Are You Getting?

There is no easy way to tell exactly how much caffeine you are getting from coffee, tea, cocoa, soft drinks, and other products. Studies and tests often add to the confusion, because the same standards are not always followed. Here's what you should know.

Beans and Leaves

Coffee. The beans make a big difference (see Chapter 2). Caffeine content varies from one coffee bean to another. Brazilian coffee has more caffeine than Colombian or Central American coffee, while Philippine coffee has more than any American coffee. And the beans used to make most popular commercial decaf coffees are higher in caffeine than those used in regular brews.

What's more, coffee beans are commodities whose prices fluctuate on world markets; blenders habitually change their blends to offset price rises in one or another kind of bean. Different blends contain different levels of caffeine.

Tea. The older the tea leaf, the more caffeine it contains. Surprisingly enough, most tea leaves have more caffeine before brewing than after. By contrast, coffee has *less* caffeine before brewing and more caffeine after—in prepared form. Only one-fourth the amount used for a coffee beverage is required to make a palatable hot tea drink. Green and black varieties and Ceylon and Indian types are highest in caffeine and sometimes in tannin as well. A South American drink, *guarana,* made from the seeds of a large woody climbing plant native to the Amazon valley, has three times as much caffeine as most coffee. It is often sold as a tea or vitamin supplement.[8]

Measuring

A cup or two of brewed coffee is generally estimated to contain 150 to 250 milligrams of coffee. But different coffees weigh different amounts—the weight of a level tablespoon of coffee differed among some brands by as much as 40%. Measure for measure, a relatively lightweight "fluffy" coffee will deliver more cups per pound.

More important is the size of the measure you're told to use. A common recipe is one level tablespoon of ground coffee for each 6-ounce cup of water you pour into the pot. That was the measure recommended for the A&P whole-bean coffee. Other brands recommend a rounded tablespoon, which is almost half again as much, or even two level tablespoons. In short, some brands' labels recommend twice as much coffee as others to brew one cup of coffee.[9]

Pot and Grind

Coffee. The amount of caffeine you get also depends on the pot and the grind. The more coffee solids that are extracted by water from the beans, the more caffeine in your cup.

And the type of grind depends on the type of pot. Higher extraction increases acidity as well, and the higher the acid, the more gastric distress coffee is likely to give you.

Coffee-making methods include steeping, in which hot—not boiling—water is mixed directly with ground coffee; percolation, in which hot water is dripped through grounds; filtration, in which hot water is dripped through grounds and a filter; espresso, in which live steam and water are forced through grounds under pressure; and the use of instant-dehydrated coffee concentrate, either blown-dry or freeze-dried, which is reconstituted with hot water.

Drip methods produce a cup of coffee 50 to 120% higher in caffeine than instant, while percolated coffee generally falls somewhere in between. Turkish- or Greek-style boiled coffee and coffee made by brewing in European plunger-type coffee makers produces higher caffeine and more harmful oils and acids than conventional pots, although exact amounts have not been determined.

Tea. Similarly, beverages made from loose tea leaves tend to produce a stronger brew with more caffeine and tannins than tea-bag tea. A weak solution—Twinings English Breakfast Tea—made with a tea bag produced a 26-milligram drink, whereas leaves brewed in a more porous metal tea ball produced a 39-milligram drink. Tea brewed from loose leaves releases more caffeine than either of these methods.[10]

Brewing Time

Coffee. How you make your coffee and the cup you use make a big difference in the amount of caffeine you get. Brewing extracts more caffeine, and an increase of just five minutes in brewing time can increase caffeine by as much as 3 to 14%.[11]

As a rule of thumb, don't percolate coffee longer than six minutes, drip longer than four to five, or brew in a vacuum or espresso-type machine longer than one to three minutes. Each extra minute adds extra caffeine.

Some studies are based on a manufacturer's directions for brewing a cup of coffee or tea. In the home, some brew it strong, and some brew it weak. Some brew it for a long time, and some don't. And it is not easy to compare studies, because cup sizes vary as well.

Dr. Alan W. Burg, a senior biochemist at Arthur D. Little Co., Cambridge, Massachusetts, reviewed the scientific literature on coffee and caffeine content and, noting the discrepancies of the National Coffee Association, suggests that 5 ounces (150 milliliters) be considered the average size of a cup.

Basing his data on twenty-nine coffee and thirteen tea products, he suggests there is an average of 85 milligrams of caffeine in a 5-ounce cup of percolated roasted ground coffee, 60 milligrams in instant coffee, and 3 milligrams in decaffeinated coffee. In actuality, the range is 64 to 124 milligrams of caffeine in percolated coffee, 40 to 108 milligrams in instant coffee, and 2 to 5 milligrams in decaffeinated coffee.

On the other hand, the Addiction Research Foundation of Ontario, Canada, which did a caffeine study based on forty-six home-brewed coffee samples and thirty-seven tea samples (some with cream or lighteners), came up with these findings: percolated coffee, 39 to 168 milligrams per cup, with 74 as the median; drip or filtered coffee, 56 to 176 milligrams, with 112 as the median; instant regular coffee, 29 to 117 milligrams, with 66 as the median; and decaffeinated coffee, 1 to 2 milligrams.[12]

Tea. As a prepared drink, tea usually has much less caffeine than coffee. But steeping time can make the caffeine count steeper.[13]

For example, a 6-ounce cup of Lipton tea contains 25 milligrams of caffeine if the strength is weak and 63 milligrams if the strength is medium. A cup of tea brewed five minutes may contain as much caffeine as a cup of instant coffee or a can of cola.

Using the same guides cited above for coffee, the National Coffee Association reports finding an average of 30 milligrams of caffeine in instant tea, with a range of 42 milligrams for bagged tea, 30 to 48 milligrams in leaf tea, and 24 to 131 milligrams in instant. The Canadian Addiction

Research Foundation showed 8 to 91 milligrams of caffeine in tea, with 27 milligrams as the median.

Roasting

Just as important as the length of brewing is the length of roasting. Longer roasting time produces darker, oilier beans. Each affects the amount of volatile oils and harsh acids released into your cup, just as longer brewing affects the release of caffeine. Thus oils may be as health-hazardous as caffeine. Although there is no standardization of grades, there *are* generally accepted categories characterized by the color of the roasted beans, the amount of oil released by the process, and the resulting flavor of the coffee brewed.[14]

Various roasts range from what coffee roasters call "light city," a cinnamon-colored roast with minimal amounts of oil, and Brazilian roast, with only a trace of oil on the surface, to the very dark, very oily roasts, such as French, Spanish, and Italian/espresso. These dark roasts should be absolutely avoided by anyone with gastrointestinal problems.

Cup Sizes

A 5- or 6-ounce cup is considered "standard" by statistics, but not in actual practice. It's preferable to think in terms of ounces, not number of cups you take in, to get a reliable estimate of your daily intake. Here's why:

1. Tea and coffee mugs for home and commercial use vary considerably in their holding capacities.

2. An after-dinner demitasse holds about 4 to 5 ounces or possibly only 3. So does an Oriental-type tea cup.

3. American tea cups, on the other hand, are likelier to hold 6 ounces.

4. Common household mugs hold about 8 ounces. But a

super mug may have a capacity of 10, 15, or even 20 ounces of coffee.

How much are you getting per serving? Just multiply the number of milligrams of caffeine per ounce given in Table 17 by the number of ounces you drink.

How Much Caffeine Are You Getting?

Fill in the blanks in Table 18 and multiply. Add the figures in the last column to get your daily caffeine dosage. Keep tabs on your intake for a week to get a good idea of how bad a habit you've got. Once you've established your intake, you can judge what your caffeine profile is:

1. *300 milligrams or more daily:* You may have a mental and physical dependency. There is nearly twice the risk of ulcers and fibrocystic disease at this level.

2. *600 milligrams or more daily:* You are almost certainly addicted to caffeine. And your risk of a heart attack at this level is almost double.

3. *1,000 milligrams or more daily:* You are really hooked and are probably unwilling or unable to kick the habit. The danger of heart disease, mental illness, cancer, or ulcers is very high. Seek help.

Table 17. Caffeine Content According to Brewing Method

Brewing method	Mg. caffeine per oz. (average)
Nonautomatic dripolator	30.2
Automatic dripolator	28.4
Nonautomatic percolator	21.4
Automatic percolator	20.8
Instant	13.2

Table 18. Caffeine Count

Product	No. cups, cans, or tablets	Mg. caffeine in each	Total mg.
Coffee (6-oz. cup)			
Regular	— ×	85	—
Instant	— ×	60	—
Decaffeinated	— ×	3	—
Reduced-caffeine beverage	— ×	20	—
		Coffee subtotal __ mg. caffeine	
Tea (6-oz. cup)			
Regular	— ×	40	—
Instant	— ×	30	—
Decaffeinated	— ×	2	—
		Tea subtotal __ mg. caffeine	
Soft drink (12-oz. can)			
Cola or pepper drink	— ×	50	—
		Soft-drink subtotal __ mg. caffeine	
Cocoa and Chocolate			
Cocoa or hot chocolate (6-oz. cup)	— ×	20	—
Chocolate candy (1 average bar)	— ×	20	—
		Cocoa and Chocolate subtotal __ mg. caffeine	
Drug (1 tablet)			
Stimulant or diet pill	— ×	100	—
Pain reliever (e.g., Vanquish, Excedrin)	— ×	65	—

163

Table 18. (Continued)

Product	No. cups, cans, or tablets		Mg. caffeine in each	Total mg.
Other analgesic (e.g., Midol, Anacin)	—	×	35	—
Cold allergy relief	—	×	30	—
Prescription medication and others	—	×	7	—
			Drug subtotal __ mg. caffeine	
			Grand total __ mg. caffeine	

SOURCES: Approximate amounts based on information supplied by the International Coffee Organization, National Coffee Association, Consumers Union, and Chocolate Manufacturers Association.

Chapter 10

Alternatives

It's obvious we could, as a nation, quit using caffeine if we cared to, or at least cut back drastically. We've done it before.

In 1946 our per capita average was 1,000 6-ounce cups. By 1979 it had declined to less than 500, largely because of cost and public knowledge about the hazards. The cost factor is gone, but we still have all the motivation we need to quit. There's convincing evidence that excessive caffeine makes us sick, tired, and addicted.

If you want to try giving it up, first find out how big a problem you've got, then ask yourself whether you want to quit or cut back, and go to it.

First the test. Then the ten-step program for caffeine quitters and reducers. Next, maintenance tips.

Is caffeine a bad habit, a very bad habit, or an addiction for you? Rate yourself. A "yes" to three to five of the questions calls for cutting back. If you answer "yes" to more than five of the following questions, chances are you are hooked on caffeine. It is a physical addiction and a psychological crutch. And you should consider quitting.

Caffeine-Users Quiz

1. Being hooked on coffee is not necessarily a simple numbers game. Drinking four to six cups of coffee a day, or even eight cups a day, does not automatically mean you're a coffee addict. Nor does one cup mean you *aren't. Are you so dependent on coffee that coffee drinking causes physical or psychological changes in your health?*
Yes __. No __.

2. Keep tabs on your intake (see Chapter 9). Ten percent of the population consumes 1 gram a day, three times the amount considered hazardous. This is certainly addictive. Anything ranging from 200 to 750 milligrams of caffeine may be a danger point at which you are likely to experience caffeinism or caffeine overdose. Pharmacologists consider amounts above 250 milligrams as large. Its effect on different people is described by many researchers as the "critical point" separating safe from excessive use. It may also be what separates safe from addictive use. In general, two to three cups of coffee per day is about what a healthy system can safely tolerate. More spells trouble. *Do you consume more than 250 milligrams every day?*
Yes __. No __.

More than 300 milligrams a day?
Yes __. No __.

3. Do you experience more than two of the recognized symptoms of caffeinism on regularly drinking one or more cups of coffee? The more you have, the likelier it is you're

hooked. The symptoms include insomnia, irritability, depression, chronic fatigue, rapid pulse or heartbeat, jitteriness, lightheadedness, rapid breathing, diarrhea, stomach pains or heartburn, headaches, and anxiety.
Yes ___. No ___.

4. *Can you start the day without a cup of coffee?*
Yes ___. No ___.

5. *Does it bother you if you ever miss your mid-morning coffee break?* And does it seem as if something's missing? Do you make up for it by having twice as much coffee later?
Yes ___. No ___.

6. *Do you usually have a second cup?*
Yes ___. No ___.

7. *Have you ever voluntarily gone a whole day without coffee or caffeinated soda or other caffeinated food and drink?* Did you feel dramatically different? Did you drink more coffee the following day?
Yes ___. No ___.

8. *Do you get headaches when you try to stop for more than 18 to 24 hours?* A Sunday-morning headache is the classic example of the addictive effects of caffeine. Breaking the routine of drinking coffee at an early hour on Friday and not resuming until Sunday causes the "caffeine withdrawal."[1]
Yes ___. No ___.

9. *Do you always choose a coffee, tea, or cola drink that has caffeine, rather than one that doesn't?*
Yes ___. No ___.

10. Do you depend on coffee every day to feel good?
Yes ___. No ___.

Ten-Step Program for Kicking the Caffeine Habit

1. The best way to withdraw from caffeine is slowly. Tapering off may be accomplished by reducing intake one cup a day over a period of a week or more.[2] If you drink a lot of coffee, abrupt withdrawal, says Dr. Morris A. Shorofsky of the Beth Israel Hospital in New York, can cause severe headaches, nausea, vomiting, and mental depression. Symptoms begin 12 to 24 hours after the last dose of caffeine.

2. Prepare yourself for pain. Coffee is a systemic poison, so doing without it will involve withdrawal symptoms. Many of these are similar to the side effects of caffeine consumption itself—yawning, drowsiness, irritability, nausea, nervousness, depression, and even a runny nose.

Withdrawal headache may be the worst part of kicking the habit, because caffeine constricts painfully dilated blood vessels in the head. "Caffeine withdrawal blahs" are nothing to worry about. They will disappear spontaneously as the sensitivity to adenosine (see page 8) returns to normal.

But don't give up, or give in. Once you've kicked the habit, you're not likely to return to coffee in any guise, say quitters who say they felt 1,000% better in just two weeks, and that the craving was gone in six weeks.

3. Discuss your desire to quit with your doctor. Half the country's M.D.'s drink no more than one or two cups daily, and 17% never touch the stuff. If he's *still* a drinker, consult a nutritionist instead—or an orthomolecular physician who understands caffeine addiction. The Academy of Preventive Medicine will supply you with references for your area.*

4. Heavy coffee drinkers are three times as likely to smoke as nondrinkers. If you're dependent on pills, alcohol, or cigarettes, along with caffeine, quitting is tougher. The medical profession calls this cross-addiction. If it's your problem, you may need outside help in quitting.[3]

5. If your efforts to quit aren't working, consult an allergist. Coffee allergy is the second severest food allergy in the country for adults. Over half of food-sensitive individuals tested have a coffee-bean intolerance. Instant coffee and tea also contain corn, another one of the worst food allergens. This could explain your addiction, and provide a professional with a key to a cure. Consult the Human Ecology Action League for names of nutritionally oriented allergists in your area.

6. Erasing your coffee-taste memory may be a gentler, slower way to quit. Drink your coffee lighter and lighter. It will help you make a transition from high-stress coffee to milk, which is rich in stress-protective nutrients, such as calcium, magnesium, and amino acids.

7. Paraphernalia can be a comfort or a trap. Don't dump your pot and your mug if they're a comfort. Just put something healthier in them and keep perking along. But if removing *all* temptation is better than trying to resist it, get rid of everything that reminds you of your habit—including commuter cups, mugs, carafes, and auto coffee-cup trays. Serve your company herbal tea or Perrier instead of the "usual." And use your supply of coffee filters for packing and mailing Christmas cookies.

* International Academy of Preventive Medicine, 34 Corporate Woods, Suite 469, 10950 Grandview, Overland Park, Kansas 66210.

8. Drink plenty of nonstimulating liquids while you're quitting—plain water, herbal tea, club soda, plain bouillon, fruit juices. You'll be orally gratified, if not coffee-fulfilled. Of those who quit coffee, 37% switch to tea. In order of popularity, the rest of the quitters turn to water (23%), nothing (14%), coffee substitutes (9%), or soft drinks, milk, or orange juice (together, 4½%). (See *Alternatives* for more suggestions.)

9. Remember coffee drinking is a conditioned reflex, too. Break the pattern by changing your automatic daily routine. Stay away from the office coffee machine and coffee shops. Walk to work. Better yet, take a vacation if you can, and break the habit while you're relaxed and away from your usual routines. Keep your hands and your mind occupied. Substitutes for picking up a coffee cup include gardening, knitting, doodling, or jumping rope, if you're house-bound. Or teach yourself solitaire. There are twenty-four variations on the game—enough to get you through the no-coffee crisis period, which lasts four to six weeks.

10. Fortify yourself physically with vitamins, which are foods, not drugs, and are nontoxic and water-soluble. You can relieve withdrawal symptoms by taking 1 gram of vitamin C every day, 500 milligrams each of B-6, B-3, and B-5, and 1 gram of calcium and 500 milligrams of magnesium. These are tranquilizers. A teaspoon of granular lecithin with meals is a nerve relaxant, or try half a teaspoon of the amino acid L-tryptophan in powdered form stirred into juice with each meal. These nutrients are more effective if taken in a timed-release form, or taken at a dosage of 100 to 500 milligrams at established intervals.

Ten-Step Caffeine-Free Maintenance Plan

1. Bad coffee substitutes will send you right back to your bad habit. If you have a connoisseur's coffee palate, don't try to wean yourself on supermarket brands. Choose a premium decaf—freeze-dried, if you like instant, or go to a coffee retail shop for fresh decaf beans and grounds, if you use regular. The flavor in both cases is usually so much better that you could mistake it for the real thing.

2. Reward yourself with something you've always wanted. After all, you'll be richer and thinner in a year. If you drink five cups a day with sugar, quitting means you save enough calories to lose at least 17 pounds in one year—more, if you drink your coffee with cream. And you'll save roughly $800 if you have a two to three-cup-a-day habit.

3. If you switch to decaf and you still feel switched off, switch to a coffee-free grain brew instead. Even decaf contains chlorogenic acid, say researchers. It's a chemical that burns up B-1 (the energy vitamin) in your system. (See section "Caffeine-Free Coffees, Teas, Colas, and Cocoas to Make and Buy" on page 173.)

4. If the going gets tough, exercise. Studies by Mary B. Harris of the University of New Mexico at Albuquerque indicate that "running seems to be associated with reduced smoking, drinking and other bad habits."

5. Maintain your caffeine-teetotaling profile while traveling by keeping herbal tea bags in your briefcase or purse so you can order hot water and do it yourself in restaurants.

6. Carry a thermos of herbal tea at all times in your car, so you won't be tempted to brake for coffee breaks. Try a combination of herbs to detoxify your system and speed up recovery. At San Francisco's Walden House Drug Rehabilitation Center, they use comfrey root, mullein, spearmint, rose hips, orange peel, and golden seal. You can get them all from any health food store and use them to make a craving-control beverage. (Use one part of golden seal to eight parts of everything else, and sip throughout the day.)

7. Dynamic imaging—a self-help technique—helps. Every time you turn down a cup, remind yourself of the ways you've benefited—caffeine has been linked for example to decreased fertility in men and birth defects—and since physical fitness is associated with a low normal resting heart rate and physical training lowers the resting heart rate in terms of the heart, caffeine can be considered an antifitness drug. Stopping coffee and tea often causes a decrease of 20 beats per minute in the resting heart rate.[4]

And coffee drinkers also have a 72% greater chance of developing ulcers, compared to nonusers. Make a list, and carry it with you.

8. Look into a behavior modification program. What works to change compulsive eating and alcohol abuse can work for a compulsive coffee-drinking habit, too.

Send for the helpful hints pamphlets available from Alcoholics Anonymous, Weight Watchers, and Smoke-Enders programs.

9. Seek out people who share your desire to quit. Talk it over with them. The companionship of other quitters will keep you motivated. They'll encourage you, not put you down.

10. A vegetarian's diet helps reduce the acid balance in the body that contributes to a craving for addictive substances. Write The Vegetarian Society of America, P.O. Box 68, Maplewood, New Jersey 07040, for more information.

Caffeine-Free Coffees, Teas, Colas, and Cocoas to Make and Buy

Quitting or cutting down?

You don't even have to give up your cup—just fill it with something else. Here are some caffeine-free suggestions to make or buy that will help you break away from your coffee, tea, or cola break.

Coffee Substitutes to Make or Buy

1. Are you a fairly heavy habitual coffee drinker? Wean yourself with a compromise—one of the new blends combining coffee beans and caffeine-free grains. Manor House Lite Coffee, for example, has one-third the caffeine of regular brew, but more of a kick than decaf. (Mix a blend half and half with decaf, and you'll lower the caffeine level to only 15%.)

2. Make Old-Fashioned Toast Coffee: Oven-toast a slice of bread to a dark brown color. Put it in a small saucepan. Pour a cup of boiling water over it. Cover and let simmer for about a minute. Press the liquid out of the toast with the back of a spoon. You now have a rich brown cup of cheer. Add milk for sweetness, or drink it as a bouillon with a dab of butter.

3. Like barley? You'll like Wilson's Heritage, the barley substitute you brew like coffee, made by The Wilson Company in Parsons, Kansas (in filter bags or 1-pound bags). It's even milder than decaf, and barley is a good nondairy source of calcium.

4. Oral gratification? Get it *without* caffeine from Postum, a tasty instant drink made only from bran, wheat, and molasses. Only 12 calories per cup, and even the kids can drink it. Available everywhere.

173

5. Chicory root and dandelion root are two of man's oldest natural no-caffeine brews. Rich in B vitamins and minerals, you can find them in all health food shops and coffee retail stores. Or send for flavored tisane teas made of natural plants and herbs. Tisane leaves have not been processed and will keep their potency and flavor longer than other tea leaves. Nine flavors packaged loose in 16-ounce apothecary jars or 2-ounce boxes are available from Josephine, Inc., 38 East Sycamore St., Box 249, Columbus, Ohio 43216. Another one is Bambu Instant made from chicory, figs, wheat, barley, and acorns in powders, packets, and a Bambu Regular grind for brewing, available from Bioforce of America Ltd., 21 West Mall, Plainview, New York 11803. (They also make an aromatic alpine tea worth stocking.)

6. *Corn Coffee:* Roast kernels of whole corn in the oven at 200 degrees until brown all the way through. Put through coffee grinder, or crush in food chopper. Can be pounded in mortar or crushed with rolling pin. Boil or perk to desired strength.

Corn meal can be roasted the same way. Place thin layer on cookie sheet and stir frequently until it looks like ground coffee. Proportion: about one tablespoon per cup.

7. Make *Half Decaf I* (only 32% caffeine per cup): mix decaf instant and regular instant coffee. Prepare as usual. Or make *Half Decaf II* (5% caffeine per cup): Mix one part of any commercial low-caffeine coffee blend—such as Sunrise or Manor House Lite—with one part no-caffeine "coffee" substitute, such as Pero or Postum. Perk as usual.

8. Sanka is *still* 2% caffeine. *Nature's Sanka* isn't. Here's a 5-minute formula: combine 2 tablespoons blackstrap molasses (a good source of the B vitamins, which coffee depletes) with ¼ teaspoon ginger. Slowly add 1½

cups water. Boil for 1 minute. Drink warm with milk or cream.

9. According to experts, the flavor of decaffeinated coffee is improved by use of a Melior pot, although the Melitta and several other drip coffee makers produce equally satisfactory conventional coffee. And for the lustiest decaffeinated coffee, order a darker roasted decaf bean.

10. Cafe Altura is an organic-gourmet coffee made from mild arabica beans. Available in light or dark roasts in preground, 12-ounce vacuum-packed cans from Terra Nova Trading Co., 717 East Ojai Ave., Ojai, California 93023. Or try The Natural Coffee, a decaf available from Au Natural, 320 Artist Rd., Santa Fe, New Mexico 87501.

11. The Miss Figgy brand is pure fig extract. Use it as a natural sweetener or as a coffee extract substitute. Rombout's, a European brand (since 1896), is an extra-mild, low-acid, water-processed decaf.

12. Put Pero in your cup. It is a no-coffee-bean and caffeine-free cereal-grain instant imported from Germany. Tastes "coffier" than decaf, and all health food stores and chains, including the national General Nutrition Corporation chain of stores, carry it.

13. Use a noncoffee bean to make your morning brew. *Beans 'n Berries Brew:*

½ cup whole or cracked soybeans*
2 cups whole rye berries*
2 cookie sheets

Soak grains and beans overnight to soften. Drain and rinse. Spread the beans on one cookie sheet, and the rye

---

* Available at all health food stores, or from natural food suppliers such as Walnut Acres, Penns Creek, Pennsylvania 17862.

berries on a second sheet. Bake beans and berries at 200 degrees for a minimum of two hours, stirring occasionally. When beans and berries are dark brown, grind them in a blender or foodmill to a cornmeal-like consistency. To brew, use 1 tablespoon of grounds for each pint of water or to taste. For added strength, add a pinch of dandelion root or chicory grounds (two more healthy coffee substitutes).

14. A more flavorful cup? To make any no-caffeine brew taste more like the real thing, put a vanilla bean into the machine when you perk. Or add a dash of soy sauce to the grounds you perk.

15. Heavy consumption of coffee can reduce your vitamin B-1 level by as much as 50% (for tea, it is 60%). Three B-vitamin-rich alternatives that don't:

- *Breakfast Cup* from Loma Linda Foods of Riverside, California.
- *Breakaway* from Celestial Seasonings, a blend made from roasted barley, roasted carob, roasted chicory root, cinnamon, dates, and natural flavors and spices. It also comes in Orange Cappuccino, Carob Mint, and Cinnamon Splendor flavors.
- Terra Nova's *Cafe Libra* water-processed decaf in vacuum-sealed cans.

16. Of moderate coffee drinkers, 54% report fatigue and tension. Energize with *miso,* a soybean extract that's restful, low in sodium, and high in pleasure and potassium. Miso-Cup is available from Edward & Sons Trading Company, Box 271, Union, New Jersey 07083, if it's not in your favorite health food store.

17. Alvita Products in Huntington Beach, California, makes another completely caffeine-free beverage called No-Kafe, which is an instant drink and is made from roasted barley, malt, roasted chicory root, and rye. Or, consider Herb Hunter's Cevada Cereal Coffee, said to be one of South America's most popular hot *and* cold coffee substitutes. And Nature's Sunshine's (a division of Amtec Industries, Spanish Fork, Utah) Herbal Beverage is a blend of roasted barley, malt, chicory, rye, and herbal flavorings.

18. An espresso alternative? Gourmets love Copenhagen Decaffeinated, available ground or in beans from White Coffee Corporation, P.O. Box 1092, Long Island City, New York 11101.

Tea Substitutes to Make or Buy

1. Satisfy your tea-zone with decaffeinated tea. Bencheley Teas, 514–516 Bay Avenue, Point Pleasant Beach, New Jersey 08742, makes six flavors, including decaffeinated Earl Grey and caffeine-free orange pekoe. Or look for the Boston Tea Company's decaf at selected supermarkets or by mail.

2. What makes a good counterfeit cup of black pekoe? Try a little potassium-rich fig or prune juice stirred into hot water. As a bonus, dried fruit juices help keep you regular and help fight the acid condition in the body that often creates a craving for caffeine, says drug researcher Dr. A. James Fixx of the University of Nebraska Medical Center.

3. Herbal teas to try in your supermarket? Look for Lipton's decaffeinated herbal teas in Flo-thru Tea Bags (flavors include Almond Pleasure and Quietly Chamomile) at most supermarkets. Many also carry the Bromley line of decaffeinated teas (Eastern Tea Corporation). And if you've had Celestial Seasonings and Twinings, try Bigelow. Or ask at your health food store.

4. Allergic to herb teas? Try a plain salt-free consommé or bouillon. Lemon juice adds an extra perk. Or try the new mocha java substitute made from extracts of the dahlia tuber. In packets at health food stores, or write Dacopa Foods, Cal Natural Products, Box 139, Manteca, California 95336.

5. A stimulant-free tea serves as a coffee, too—try Celestial Seasonings's Roastaroma, a blend of roasted barley, crystal malt, roasted chicory root, roasted carob, cassia bark, allspice, and star anise. It comes loose, to perk like coffee, and in bags to brew for tea.

6. Make yourself some *Solar Decaf:* In a clear glass, half-gallon jar, place five herbal tea bags (or decaf tea bags), and fill the jar with cold water. Put the lid on and set the jar in the sun outside or in a very sunny window. In a couple of hours the tea will have reached the right color. Remove the tea bags and chill the tea. Makes eight cups.

7. Make *Fruit and Fiber Tea* (it's naturally sweetened):

15 chopped raisins
3 tablespoons bran
1 pint boiling water

Soak raisins and bran for 8 hours in the boiling water. Strain and drink hot or cold. Very high in iron. Serves two.

8. Make caffeine-free iced tea: Iced tea connoisseurs say one of the best herbs for the purpose is linden (or lime flower), lemon balm (or lovage), or borage. All are reputed to increase the coldness of any liquid in which they are steeped.

9. Spices are nice no-caffeine stimulants. A cup of ginger tea stimulates, as does cayenne without caffeine. Or look for the spicy-flavored Mu Tea, a blend sold at all health food stores.

10. Reduce the danger in your cup by adding cream (not

lemon juice) to your cup to decrease the tannin content. Tannins cause gastrointestinal disorders, and may be weak carcinogens.

Sources for Coffee and Tea Substitutes

If your health food store or local coffee and tea merchant can't give you what you want, write the following mail order suppliers. Request a catalog.

American Tea, Coffee and Spice Company, 1511 Champa St., Denver, Colorado 80202

Caravansary, 2263 Chestnut St., San Francisco, California 94123

The Coffee Bean, Burlington Mall, 777 Guelph Line, Burlington, Ontario, Canada

The Coffee Bean, 13020-D San Vincente Blvd., Los Angeles, California 90049

The Coffee Trader, 2619 North Downer Ave., Milwaukee, Wisconsin 53211

Empire Coffee and Tea Company, 486 Ninth Ave., New York, New York 10018

Zabar's, 2245 Broadway, New York, New York 10024

The Sensuous Bean, 228 Columbus Ave., New York, New York 10023

McNulty's Tea and Coffee Company, 109 Christopher St., New York, New York 10014

The Schapira Coffee Company, 117 West 10th St., New York, New York 10011

Walnut Acres, Penns Creek, Pennsylvania 17862

Aphrodisia, 282 Bleecker St., New York, New York 10014

D'Amico Foods, 309 Court St., Brooklyn, New York 11231

Caffeine-Free Colas to Make or Buy

1. Why join the Pepsi generation? Make *Black Pekoe Cola:* Combine cold brewed decaffeinated black pekoe tea with seltzer or club soda. Sweeten. Serve with orange slivers.

2. Worthington Foods of Loma Linda, California, makes Caffree Cola. Available in six-pack cans at your health food store.

3. Make *Vita Cola:* Fill a saucepan with fresh, dark purple grapes and an inch of water. Cover and bring to a boil, then simmer just until the skins begin to burst, not more than a few minutes. Strain, and press the grapes through a sieve to leave the skins and seeds behind. Stir in sweetener and lemon juice to taste. Chill. Serve diluted with water or club soda to your taste. Add 1 tablespoon grape or cherry concentrate for a thicker, heavier soda taste.

4. Buy a soda siphon and make your own counterfeit cola. Soda siphons turn plain water into seltzer, save money, and excite kids. All you do is fill the one-quart container with tap water, insert a carbon dioxide cartridge at the top, and out comes the salt-free seltzer. Combine with natural caramel syrup, and you are in business.

The siphon costs about $56. One source is Hammacher Schlemmer, 145 East 57th St., New York, New York 10022. (212) 421-9000.

5. How about a *Mr. Pepper-Upper* of your own?

Combine 2 cups apple juice, 2 cups peppermint or spearmint tea, ½ cup cold Perrier water, and ½ teaspoon white pepper (a flavor enhancer). Shake well. Serve over frozen lemon-spiked ice cubes, or with fresh lemon curls.

6. Here's a new use for *gotu kola,* a naturally stimulating herb similar to ginseng that's widely used in the Orient.

Combine cold brewed *gotu-kola* herbal tea with two parts plain, carbonated water. Sweeten with honey. Garnish with lemon peel.

7. *Fructose Fruit Soda:*

½ cup each cold orange juice, water, pineapple juice
1 large peach, peeled, chopped
   Pinch nutmeg

Put all ingredients in a blender and whirl until smooth. Dilute as desired with water or sparkling water. (The fructose in fruits is a pick-me-up. Unlike caffeine, it does not damage the nervous system.)

8. *Valley Dew:*

½ cup honey
2 cups water
   Grated rind of 1 lemon
1 cup fresh lemon juice

Dissolve honey in water over high flame, stirring constantly. Boil 2 to 3 minutes while stirring. Remove from heat, and add lemon rind and juice. Freeze until mixture begins to thicken. Stir with fork. Repeat this procedure until ice pellets form. Spoon into glasses. Add carbonated water to taste. *Variation:* Substitute 1 cup unsweetened white grape juice (Welch's makes one) for lemon juice.

9. *Power Pop:*

1½ cups orange juice
½ cup cranberry juice
2 tablespoons lemon juice
2 tablespoons honey
1 pint sparkling water
½ teaspoon angostura bitters

Blend juices and honey. Add carbonated water and angostura bitters. Freeze half to make un-Pepsi cubes to pop into other homemade soda pops.

10. *Sugar-Free Caffeine-Free Diet Cola:*

4 tablespoons black cherry concentrate, undiluted
1 teaspoon lemon juice
1 cup club soda or sparkling water
Ice cubes or crushed ice chips
Orange slices

In tall glass, mix concentrate, lemon juice, and soda. Add ice, and garnish with orange slices. Makes one serving. About 45 calories per serving. (Natural fruit concentrates are carried by most health food stores—or substitute undiluted grape juice concentrate.)

11. What hits the spot better than Pepsi and provides natural vitamin C? *Herbal Cola:* Turn any dark, spicy herbal tea (mu, rose hip, or raspberry leaf) into a cola substitute. Sweeten, chill, combine with sparkling water, and serve over shaved ice. A twist of lemon heightens flavor.

12. Make your own *High-C Cola:* Combine an ascorbic acid-rich herbal tea—rose hip, acerola berry, persimmon, lemon balm, or nettle—with a little vitamin C-rich citrus juice. Add carbonated water, swizzle, and sip.

13. Caffeine-free colas—sweetened with honey or fructose—are manufactured by Health Valley, Rich Life, and Hansen Brands. Ask at your health food store for these and other brands, also available in gourmet shops and many supermarkets.

14. Fruit "drinks" aren't good cola substitutes. There are six teaspoons of sugar in a single glass, says Dr. Abraham E. Nizel, professor of oral health services at the Tufts University School of Medicine—enough to produce 20 to

30 minutes' worth of decay-causing acid. To make a healthy homemade juice drink, combine one part pure juice with eight parts water, and sweeten to taste.

Caffeine-Free Hot Chocolate and Cocoa Drinks to Make or Buy

1. Moo-Hoo (the brown cow alternative): Process 1 tablespoon light molasses and ½ teaspoon cinnamon with 2 cups milk in blender. Chill.

2. Cow Punch (the Yoohoo alternative): Combine 1 teaspoon blackstrap molasses and 1 teaspoon unsweetened carob powder with 16 ounces warm milk. Shake vigorously. Chill. (Carob powder is available at health food stores and some gourmet shops and supermarkets.)

3. Caffeine-Free Cocoa:

1 cup milk
2 tablespoons carob powder
1 slice ginger root, chopped into small pieces
2 tablespoons honey

Heat carob milk (carob powder is available in health food stores and some supermarkets) and ginger slowly and gently for 10 minutes. Do not boil. Strain and add honey. Drink warm or chilled. VARIATIONS: Substitute buttermilk for carob milk. For milder drink, reduce amount of ginger or eliminate.

4. Sugar-free carob, a natural cocoa and chocolate alternative, is available in powder, bar, and chip forms at all health food stores and in the health food section of some supermarkets. Or write El Molino Mills, P.O. Box 2156, 345 North Baldwin Park Boulevard, City of Industry, California 91746.

5. If you're chock full of cocoa, you're chock full of caffeine, too: there's 50 milligrams in cocoa, a third as much in hot chocolate. Switch to the grains-figs-and-acorns-based Bambu, still made according to the original formula of the famous Swiss naturopath, Alfred Vogel. It has a realistic flavor that is rich and full-bodied. Available in instant or regular brewable form at health food stores and better supermarkets.

Twenty-Five Ways to Consume Less Caffeine

1. Switch your coffee-making method. Brewed coffee contains twice the caffeine of instant. And drip produces higher caffeine levels than percolated. New light "blends" or decafs are lowest. Brewing tea for 1 minute rather than 5 reduces caffeine by 50%.

2. Cut down by mixing your regular coffee with decaf. By gradually increasing the decaf and decreasing the regular, you'll make a total switch. (Other hints on "healthy adulteration" in recipe section.)

3. Reduce the number of cups or cans of coffee, tea, or soda you drink in a day. "Caffeine is a far more effective stimulant if it is used infrequently," says *New York Times* health reporter Jane Brody. One cup is also a lot safer than three—the level at which ulcers and birth defects have been noted.

4. Caffeine and tannin are what give regular tea its bite. If herbal substitutes taste "wishy-washy," flavor with additional herbs, such as mint, lemon, balm, grated ginger, lemon juice, or anise seed.

5. Tempted to go for seconds? Have water instead. It fills you up and even supplies minerals, such as calcium, zinc, and copper.

6. Had your wake-up cup? Buy one for the road, but only drink half.

7. Be alive at five *without* using up a day's supply of adrenalin. Bee pollen tablets contain sixteen vitamins, sixteen minerals, eighteen amino acids, eighteen enzymes, and twenty-eight trace elements—all help to lift and stabilize your energy levels. Studies reveal that athletes in training who take bee pollen daily recover their energy faster after exercise and fatigue.

8. Switch to beans with less caffeine. The three varieties of coffee beans with the *lowest* caffeine content (1.13%) are Santos, Minas, and Ethiopian Mocca. The two coffee beans containing the *most* (2.30%) are Robusta Congo and Robusta Uganda. Guatemala and Salvador, two varieties popular in the United States, are in the middle, with 1.32%.

9. Instead of making coffee in the morning, make love, do the laundry, walk the dog, or just get up too late to plug in the pot.

10. Change your coffee break time. According to Dr. Charles Ehret, a researcher at the Argonne National Laboratory in Chicago, coffee for breakfast slows you down during the day and stirs you up at night. If you've got to have a cup, have it at 3:30 or 4 o'clock in the afternoon. At that point, the effect is neutral; it neither advances nor delays the metabolic cycle.

11. What works to beat a nicotine habit often helps caffeine addiction. Write for a copy of Clearing the Air, a handy book filled with useful tips put out by the National Cancer Institute, 777 Third Ave., New York, New York 10017.

12. Replace wake-up coffee with a workout. Walking conditions the entire cardiovascular system. All the body's organs benefit. Even your kidneys get a hand from your

moving feet. An acupuncture point located just behind the ankle bone relates to kidney function; stimulating the point aids in the breakdown and removal of uric acid, which is built up in the blood by caffeine, and which causes sluggishness of both the mind and the body.

13. Don't drink, doodle. According to Dr. Stephen Brown, associate professor of psychology at Pepperdine University in Los Angeles, California, "Doodling and carefree drawing releases the cork on bottled-up stress and tension . . . it restores vitality and health through relaxation. Everyone can really erase stress by doodling." For full effect, a doodle break should last 15 minutes.

14. Increase exercise. According to Robert Rodale, head of the Soil and Health Society, "The more active you are physically, the more you turn to water instead of stimulating or intoxicating drinks for your beverage needs. Physical activity makes us feel good in ways far better and more effective than any kind of drugs . . . such as caffeine. Anyone who turns to them for a long-lasting lift is in for a letdown. . . . I drink coffee occasionally, but only a few sips from a cup, just to get the taste. If I'm looking for a quick lift to my spirits, I'll go out and take a walk."[5]

15. The Chinese national drink is hot water and/or low-caffeine green tea at meals. It could work for you, too.[6]

16. Don't switch to cola to reduce caffeine. Studies indicate you may just drink more to get the amount of caffeine you're used to.

17. Drink less and enjoy it more. Opt for moderate self-indulgence, says food writer Raymond Sokolov, and you can drink small amounts of very good coffee. "Putting the standard two tablespoons of ground coffee into six ounces of water twice a day, you will risk little and improve the enjoyment of life through astute exploitation of a useful plant."[7]

18. Sip a safer stimulant. Good alternatives include herbal teas, such as ginseng, peppermint, ginger root, or cayenne tea (all available in capsules, too); the seaweed kelp; the plankton food spirulina; and B-vitamins niacin (B-3) and thiamine (B-1), available in tablets, help. Other healthful alternatives are the mineral magnesium and magnesium-rich foods, such as nuts and grains.

19. Two tricks for reducing caffeine and tannin in the tea you drink: don't use sugar or a tea cozy. Sugar numbs the palate and prompts you to compensate by drinking more. A cozy causes the tea to steep too long, increasing stimulant content.

20. Get your lift from vitamin C, not cola drinks. According to studies by Dr. Emmanuel Cheraskin, head of the University of Alabama's Department of Oral Medicine, taking larger doses of vitamin C (1 gram or more) makes you much less susceptible to fatigue. Vitamin C also increases resistance to infection, guards against excessive bruising, and assists in the healing of wounds.[8]

21. Take a cycling break, not a caffeine break. "Men who have bicycled vigorously for most of their lives are ten times less likely to develop heart disease then are others their age," says British physician H. K. Robertson. Lifelong cyclists over age 75 show a tenfold decrease in heart disease.

22. Carry snacks to fight your "caffeine-crazies." Raisins, small apples, carrot sticks, nuts, and chewable protein tablets from the health food store help to elevate your blood sugar levels.

23. Practice going without coffee and cola. Think of quitting in terms of one day at a time. Tell yourself you won't drink today, and then don't.

24. Make a list of things you'd like to buy yourself (or someone else). Estimate the cost in terms of cups of coffee and cans of soda, and put the money aside to buy these gifts.

25. Improve your diet. According to Alexander G. Schauss, director of the American Institute for Biosocial Research in Tacoma, Washington, "Nourishment deficiencies can produce unhealthy desires for alcohol, marijuana, tobacco, and drugs such as caffeine." A dietary deficiency of zinc can increase the desire for stimulants, says Schauss, "and reduce the taste for vegetables."[9]

Notes

Chapter 1

1. National Coffee Association, 120 Wall Street, New York, N.Y.
2. *USA Today*, May 23, 1983.
3. USDA figures, International Report, *New York Times*, July 18, 1983.
4. *Mother Earth News*, November 19, 1981.
5. Charles Wetherall, *Kicking the Coffee Habit* (Minneapolis, Minn.: Wetherall Publishing Co., 1981).
6. *Star*, November 19, 1982.
7. *Journal of the American Medical Association*, December 18, 1967.
8. Public Information Bulletin of General Nutrition Corp., Fargo, N. Dak., 1981.
9. James W. Long, *The Essential Guide to Prescription Drugs*, revised ed. (New York: Harper & Row, 1980).
10. *New York Times*, April 21, 1982, p. C6.
11. "News Digest," *Vegetarian Times*, April 1983.
12. *VIM Newsletter*, December 1979.

13. Edward M. Brecher and the editors of *Consumer Reports, Licit and Illicit Drugs: The Consumers Union Report on Narcotics, Stimulants, Depressants, Inhalants, Hallucinogens, and Marijuana—Including Caffeine, Nicotine, and Alcohol* (Mount Vernon, N.Y.: Consumers Union, 1972), p. 205.

14. Avram Goldstein and Sophia Kaizer, "Psychotropic Effects of Caffeine in Man. III. A Questionnaire Survey of Coffee Drinking and Its Effects in a Group of Housewives," Clinical Pharmacology and Therapeutics, vol. 10, July 8, 1969, p. 482.

15. Edward M. Brecher, *Licit and Illicit Drugs.*

16. U.S. Department of Agriculture, *Toxicity of Caffeine*, 1917.

17. *Nutrition Health Review*, Winter 1982, p. 5.

18. National Coffee Association, 120 Wall Street, New York, N.Y.

19. *The Runner*, January 1980.

20. Reporter Sandra Earley, Knight-Ridder Newspapers, 1981.

21. Jane Brody, *Jane Brody's Nutrition Book* (New York: Norton, 1980).

22. *New York Times*, March 16, 1983, p. C9.

23. *Mother Earth News*, July 1981, p. 146.

24. *National Enquirer*, May 5, 1981, p. 11.

25. *Journal of Applied Nutrition*, vol. 33, no. 1, 1981.

26. Tom Ferguson, in *Mother Earth News*, July 1981.

27. *East West Journal*, April 1978.

28. *Advertising Age*, February 14, 1983.

29. *Medical Self Care* magazine, 1981.

30. *New York Times,* April 21, 1982.

31. Associated Press report, December 30, 1980.

Chapter 2

1. *National Enquirer*, June 29, 1982.

2. Sanders, Girling, Davies, and Sanders, "Would You Believe," *The Healthways*, October–November 1980, p. 26.

3. *The Harvard Medical School Health Letter*, vol. 7, no. 9, June, 1982.
4. *Saturday Evening Post*, May–June 1982, p. 50.
5. *Consumer Reports*, March 1983.
6. National Coffee Association, 120 Wall St., New York, N.Y.
7. Edward M. Brecher. *Licit and Illicit Drugs.*
8. *New York Times*, March 16, 1983.
9. *Moneysworth*, March 1980.
10. National Coffee Association, 120 Wall St., New York, N.Y.
11. James Trager, *The Food Book* (New York: Avon Books, 1972).
12. *Nutrition Health Review*, Winter 1982.
13. *Ibid.*
14. *FDA Consumer*, September 1980, p. 30.
15. Lewis E. Machatka, in *Better Life Journal*, March 1981.
16. *New York* magazine, November 17, 1975.
17. Ray Josephs, in *Nutrition Health Review*, Winter 1982.
18. Carol Ann Rinzler, in *Sunday News Magazine, New York Daily News*, October 9, 1977.
19. James Trager, *The Food Book.*
20. Robert S. de Ropp, *Drugs and the Mind* (New York: St. Martin's Press–Delta Books, 1976), p. 248.
21. T. D. Crothers, *Morphinism and Narcomanias From Other Drugs* (Philadelphia: W. B. Saunders & Co., 1902).
22. *Consumer Reports*, October 1979.
23. *Ibid.*
24. Personal communication from National Coffee Association, 120 Wall St., New York, N.Y.
25. *Nutrition Action*, May 1981, p. 20.
26. *New York Times*, April 24, 1982.
27. Richard H. Zander, "Are You a Caffeine Junkie?" *Saturday Evening Post*, May–June, 1982.
28. *National Enquirer*, October 2, 1979.
29. Charles Wetherall, *Kicking the Coffee Habit.*
30. Study by Herbert Moskowitz, Insurance Institute for Highway Safety, October 1980.

31. *National Enquirer,* November 10, 1981.
32. Benjamin Kissin and Henri Begleiter, eds. *The Biology of Alcoholism,* vol. 3 (New York: Plenum Press, 1974).
33. National Coffee Association, 120 Wall St., New York, N.Y., May 1981.
34. National Breakfast Survey, 1979.
35. *Bestways,* August 1982.
36. H. L. Newbold, *Dr. Newbold's Revolutionary New Discoveries About Weight Loss* (New York: New American Library, 1977).
37. Carol Ann Rinzler, *Strictly Female* (New York: New American Library, 1981).
38. International Coffee Organization, October 1980.
39. *New York Times,* April 21, 1982, p. C6.
40. *Restaurant Business,* March 1, 1979.
41. Letter to author, February 25, 1983.
42. Kenneth Anderson, *The Pocket Guide to Coffees and Teas* (New York: Perigree Books, 1982).

Chapter 3

1. *New York Times,* August 26, 1982.
2. "Coffee Nerves," *New York,* September 13, 1982.
3. *The World Cup,* International Coffee Organization, London, England, Winter 1979.
4. Paavo Airola, *How to Get Well* (Scottsdale, Ariz.: Health Plus Publishers, 1974).
5. Paavo Airola, "Health Forum," *Vegetarian Times,* June 1982.
6. *Nutrition Health Review,* Winter 1982.
7. Edward M. Brecher, *Licit and Illicit Drugs.*
8. Charles Wetherall, *Kicking the Coffee Habit.*
9. *Nutrition Health Review,* Winter 1982.
10. *Nutrition Action,* August 1982.
11. *Nutrition Health Review,* Winter 1982.

12. *The Lancet*, 1972-II, p. 1278, 1973.
13. Charles Wetherall, *Kicking the Coffee Habit*.
14. *Current Surgery*, September–October 1980.
15. *Vegetarian Times*, July–August 1979, p. 6.
16. John Tobe, *Treasury of Natural Health Knowledge* (Provoker Press, 1973).
17. *Journal of Norwegian Medical Associates*, November 10, 1973.
18. *New York Times*, May 16, 1982, p. 47.
19. *The Health Letter*, December 10, 1982.
20. *Nutrition Action*, November 1982.
21. *Nutrition Action*, June 1982.
22. *Ibid.*
23. "How Our Coffee Is Decaffeinated," *Whole Foods*, August 1980.
24. *Better Nutrition*, April 1983.
25. *Nutrition Action*, June 1982; and *New York Times*, June 30, 1982 (Good Living section).
26. Joel Schapira, David, and Karl, *The Book of Coffee and Tea* (New York: St. Martin's Press, 1975).
27. "Dangers of Decaffeination," *Nutrition Action*, April 1982.

Chapter 4

1. Shirley Ross, *Nature's Drinks* (New York: Vintage Books, 1974), pp. 134–38.
2. Letter from Nutrition Research Dept., Kellogg Co., February 14, 1983.
3. James Trager, *The Food Book*.
4. Charles Wetherall, *Kicking the Coffee Habit*.
5. Gay Jervey, "Lipton Jumps into Fray with Decaffeinated Tea," *Advertising Age*, May 2, 1983.
6. *Health Food Business*, October 1982.
7. Kenneth Anderson, *Guide to Coffees and Teas*.
8. James Trager, *The Food Book*.

9. *Ibid.*
10. "Caffeine Used in Chemical Food Processing," *American Journal of Clinical Nutrition*, October 1978.
11. *International Journal of Vitamins and Nutrients Research*, vol. 46, 1976.
12. *Spring Magazine*, June 1982.
13. Quentin R. Regestein and James R. Rechs, *Sound Sleep* (New York: Simon & Schuster, 1980).
14. *American Journal of Clinical Nutrition*, October 1978.
15. *Tea and Coffee Trade Journal*, January 1975.
16. *The Allergy Encyclopedia*, edited by Asthma Allergy Foundation of America and Craig T. Norback (New York: New American Library, 1981).
17. *Ibid.*
18. *British Medical Journal*, vol. 282, March 1981, p. 864.
19. *Nutrition Health Review*, Winter 1982.
20. *Organic Gardening and Farming*, March 1981.
21. Donald R. Germann and Margaret Danbrot, *Anti-Cancer Diet* (New York: Wideview Books, 1977).
22. *Indian Journal of Nutrition and Dietetics*, vol. 16, no. 9, 1979.
23. *National Enquirer*, September 29, 1979.
24. *Canadian Medical Association Journal*, vol. 121, September 22, 1979, p. 6.
25. Donald R. Germann and Margaret Danbrot, *Anti-Cancer Diet.*
26. *National Enquirer*, May 3, 1976.
27. *Ibid.*
28. *National Enquirer*, September 29, 1979.
29. *Canadian Emergency Medicine*, vol. 11, October 1979, p. 10.
30. *Star Reporter*, January 20, 1981.
31. Charles Wetherall, *Kicking the Coffee Habit.*
32. *Advertising Age*, May 2, 1983.
33. *The Herbalist*, February 1979, p. 7.

34. *Nutrition Health Review*, Winter 1981.
35. *National Enquirer*, September 29, 1979.

Chapter 5

1. *Consumer Reports*, October 1981.
2. *New York Times*, March 1, 1983.
3. *Consumer Reports*, October 1981.
4. *FDA Consumer*, October 1980.
5. Cornell University News and Feature Service, February 3, 1982.
6. *National Enquirer*, May 29, 1979.
7. *New York Times*, August 26, 1983 (Business section).
8. Bureau of Industrial Economics, Washington, D.C., October 1981, report.
9. *New York Times*, March 1, 1983.
10. *Food Technology Magazine*, May–February 1981.
11. *Nutrition Action*, August 1981.
12. Center for Science in the Public Interest, *Bulletin*, June 1982.
13. Lee Smith, "The Soft Drink Wars," *Fortune Magazine*, June 30, 1980.
14. *New York Daily News*, May 25, 1983, p. 40.
15. Lawrence Dietz, *Soda Pop* (New York: Simon & Schuster, 1973).
16. *Consumer Reports*, October 1981.
17. *USA Today*, May 27, 1983, p. 1.
18. Center for Science in the Public Interest, *Bulletin*, June 1982.
19. *Beverage Industry Magazine*, September 1979.
20. *Prevention*, March 1982.
21. *New York Times*, May 28, 1981.
22. *National Enquirer*, December 16, 1979. Article by Dr. Stephan Kreitzman.
23. *Self*, June 1981.

24. *Nutrition Health Review*, Winter 1982.
25. *Nutrition Action*, August 1981.
26. Irving Wallace and David Wallechinsky, *Book of Lists #2* (New York: William Morrow & Co., 1980).
27. *Food Institute Weekly Digest*, October 8, 1980.
28. *Your Health Medical Bulletin*, February 15, 1983.
29. *Prevention*, August 1980.
30. Doris J. Rapp, in *Allergies and Your Family* (New York: Sterling Publications, 1980).
31. *Medical Tribune*, March 31, 1982.
32. *Saturday Evening Post*, May 5, 1982.
33. *The Allergy Encyclopedia.*
34. "Health News Roundup," *Health Quarterly*, October 1980, p. 67.
35. Mary Louise Bunker and Margaret McWilliams, "Caffeine Content of Common Beverages," *Journal of the American Dietetic Association*, vol. 74, January 1979.
36. Jack Alspan, in *Let's Live*, January 1981.
37. *Let's Live*, January 1981.
38. *The Star Reporter*, October 7, 1980.

Chapter 6

1. Juliette Elkon, *The Chocolate Cookbook* (New York: Bobbs-Merrill, 1973).
2. Gary Null, *How to Get Rid of the Poisons in Your Body* (New York: Arco Publishing Co., 1977).
3. *Time*, July 12, 1982.
4. *Ibid.*
5. Dr. Michael Liebowitz, in *Prevention*, September 1980.
6. *Coffee and Tea Trade Journal*, January 1975.
7. *New York Times*, December 17, 1980.
8. J. M. Ritchie, "Central Nervous System Stimulants: The Xanthines," in L. S. Boodman and A. Gilman, eds., *The Pharmacological Basis of Therapeutics*, 4th ed. (New

York: Macmillan, 1970); and E. B. Truitt, Jr., "The Xanthines," in J. R. DePalma, ed., *Drill's Pharmacology in Medicine*, 4th ed. (New York: McGraw-Hill, 1971).

9. *Let's Live*, February 1978.
10. *Nutrition Health Review*, December 1982.
11. Marcia Wilkinson, *Migraine and Headaches* (New York: Arco Publishing Co., 1982).
12. *APM Monthly Memo*, Washington, D.C., September 10, 1980.
13. Paavo Airola, "Health Forum," *Vegetarian Times*, December 1982, p. 66.
14. *Annals of Allergy,* October 1978.

Chapter 7

1. *Physicians' Desk Reference* (Oradell, N.J.: Medical Economics Co., 1982).
2. *Medical Update Magazine*, vol. 10.
3. Edward M. Brecher, *Licit and Illicit Drugs.*
4. William Philpott, in *Bestways*, May 1982.
5. *Ibid.*
6. *USA Today*, February 15, 1983.
7. S. M. Mueller and E. B. Solow, *Annals of Neurology*, vol. 11, March 1982, p. 322.
8. *Saturday Evening Post*, May 6, 1982.
9. *Nutrition Health Review*, Winter 1981.
10. *Consumer Guide to Prescription Drugs* (Publications International, May 1982).
11. Vanderbilt University Medical Center Study, *Parents Magazine*, November 1981, p. 8; and James W. Long, *The Essential Guide to Prescription Drugs.*
12. Edward M. Brecher, *Licit and Illicit Drugs.*
13. *FDA Consumer*, March 1978.
14. James W. Long, *The Essential Guide to Prescription Drugs.*

15. *Ibid.*
16. *Ibid.*
17. *Ibid.*
18. *Ibid.*
19. Donald R. Germann and Margaret Danbrot, *Anti-Cancer Diet.*
20. *National Enquirer,* September 29, 1979.

Chapter 8

1. Science Information File, March of Dime Birth Defects Foundation, September 1980.
2. *New England Journal of Medicine,* vol. 306, January 1982, p. 141.
3. *Medical World News,* April 17, 1978.
4. *Canadian Medical Journal,* September 1, 1982.
5. News release by Center for Science in the Public Interest, 1755 S St., N.W., Washington, D.C. 20006.
6. *Community Nutrition Newsletter,* April 6, 1980, p. 6.
7. *Postgraduate Medicine,* September 1977.
8. *National Enquirer,* April 29, 1980.
9. *National Enquirer,* June 2, 1981.
10. Michael Jacobson, in *Caveat Emptor,* January 1981, p. 8.
11. *New York Times,* August 28, 1982.
12. *Chimo Magazine,* June 1981.
13. Weathersbee *et al.,* in *Postgraduate Medicine,* September 1977.
14. *Ibid.*
15. Associated Press report in *New York Times,* October 19, 1982.
16. Science Information File, March of Dimes Birth Defects Foundation, September 1980.
17. R. V. Patwardhan, P. V. Desmond, Raymond F. Johnson, and Steven Schenker, "Impaired Elimination of Caffeine

by Oral Contraceptive Steroids," *Journal of Laboratory Clinical Medicine*, April 1980.

18. *Obstetrical Gynecology News*, November 1, 1977.
19. *New York Times*, January 10, 1982.
20. *New York Times*, March 12, 1981.
21. Brian MacMahon, Stella Yen, Dimitrio Trichopolous, and George Nardi, "Coffee and Cancer of the Pancreas," *New England Journal of Medicine*, March 12, 1981.
22. G. R. Howe *et al.*, "Tobacco Use, Occupation Coffee, Various Nutrients and Bladder Cancer," *Journal of the National Cancer Institute*, vol. 64, no. 4, April 1980.
23. Donald R. Germann and Margaret Danbrot, *Anti-Cancer Diet*.
24. A. S. Morrision *et al.*, *Journal of the National Cancer Institute*, vol. 68, January 1982, p. 91.
25. Donald R. Germann and Margaret Danbrot, *Anti-Cancer Diet*.
26. *Ibid.* ·
27. *Ibid.*
28. Richard H. Zander, in *Saturday Evening Post*, May–June 1982, pp. 50–54.
29. S. Heyden *et al.*, "Coffee Consumption and Mortality," *Archives of Internal Medicine*, vol. 138, October 1978.
30. S. Heyden *et al.*, "Smoking and Coffee Consumption in Three Groups: Cancer Deaths, Cardiovascular Deaths and Living Controls. A Prospective Study in Evans County, Georgia," *Journal of Chronic Diseases*, vol. 32, pp. 673–77; and O. Paul, in *Postgraduate Medicine*, vol. 44, 1968, p. 196.
31. Hershel Jick, *New England Journal of Medicine*, 1973.
32. *New England Journal of Medicine*, April 6, 1983.
33. *Medical World News*, May 1, 1978.
34. *Consumer Bulletin Annual*, 1972.
35. *New England Journal of Medicine*, vol. 298, no. 4, 1978, p. 181.
36. *Runner's World*, January 1979.

37. *Ibid.,* July 1978.
38. Richard H. Zander, in *Saturday Evening Post,* May–June 1982, pp. 50–54.
39. *Journal of Learning Disabilities,* May 1980.
40. J. F. Greden, "Coffee, Tea and You," *The Sciences,* January 1979, pp. 6–11.
41. M. T. Schwertz and G. Marbach, "Effets physiologiques de la caféine et meprobamate au cours du sommeil chez l'homme," *Arch. Sci. Physiol,* vol. 19, 1965, p. 425.
42. *National Enquirer,* August 24, 1982.
43. C. L. Anderson and S. Gates, in *Diabetologia,* 1976.
44. *The Lancet,* vol. 1, 1967, page 789.
45. *The Harvard Medical School Health Letter,* January 1981, p. 5.
46. Edward M. Brecher, *Licit and Illicit Drugs.*
47. *National Enquirer,* May 5, 1981.
48. Emmanuel Cheraskin, in *Let's Live,* June 1979.
49. S. Cohen, "Pathogenesis of Coffee-Induced Gastrointestinal Symptoms," *New England Journal of Medicine,* vol. 303, no. 3, July 17, 1980.
50. *New England Journal of Medicine,* vol. 293, 1975, pp. 897–99.
51. *Today's Nutrition,* vol. 13, no. 5, May 1982.
52. Charles Wetherall, *Kicking the Coffee Habit.*
53. *Today's Nutrition,* vol. 13, no. 5, May 1982.
54. *Journal of Drug Education,* vol. 12, no. 3, 1982.
55. Robert E. Rothenberg, *The Complete Book of Breast Care* (New York: Ballantine Books, 1975), p. 177.
56. Reported by E. K. Sanders in *Audio-Digest Obstetrics/Gynecology,* vol. 27, no. 1.
57. *Good Housekeeping,* August 1980, p. 210.
58. *New York Times,* April 21, 1982.
59. *Vegetarian Times,* July/August 1976, p. 6.
60. *Harvard Medical School Health Letter,* June 1982.
61. James Trager, *The Food Book.*
62. *Bestways,* January 1981.

63. Richard Mackarness, *Living Safely in a Polluted World* (New York: Stein and Day, 1980).
64. *New York Times*, April 21, 1982.
65. Carl C. Pfeiffer, *Brain Allergies: The Psychonutrient Connection* (New Canaan, Conn.: Keats Publishing, 1980).
66. *International Journal of Vitamin and Nutrition Research*, February 1976.
67. *Journal of Laboratory and Clinical Medicine*, January 1982.
68. Arthritis Research, P.O. Box 5688, Santa Monica, Calif., 90405.
69. *Chimo Magazine*, June 1981.
70. Lawrence Galton, *Medical Advances* (New York: Crown, 1977).

Chapter 9

1. *Physicians' Desk Reference* (Oradell, N.J.: Medical Economics, Co., 1982).
2. *Let's Live*, July 1976, p. 20.
3. *Ibid.*
4. *Ibid.*
5. James W. Long, *The Essential Guide to Prescription Drugs*.
6. *American Journal of Psychology.* Report quoted by Richard H. Zander in *Saturday Evening Post*, May-June 1982, p. 52.
7. Health, Education, and Welfare Publication no. (FDA) 78-3070.
8. James Trager, *The Food Book*.
9. *Consumer Reports*, March 1983.
10. Mary Louise Bunker and Margaret McWilliams, "Caffeine Content of Common Beverages," *Journal of the American Dietetic Association*, vol. 74, 1979.
11. Charles Wetherall, *Kicking the Coffee Habit*.

12. Technical work prepared by biochemist Alan W. Burg of Arthur D. Little, Inc., Cambridge, Mass., in 1975 for the National Coffee Association.
13. Mary Louise Bunker and Margaret McWilliams, "Caffeine Content."
14. Kenneth Anderson, *The Pocket Guide to Coffees and Teas.*

Chapter 10

1. John F. Greden, "Caffeinism: Diagnosing the Dilemma," *New England Journal of Medicine*, vol. 303, p. 4.
2. *New York Times*, January 26, 1977.
3. *New England Journal of Medicine*, January 21, 1982.
4. *New England Journal of Medicine*, vol. 308, 1983, p. 814.
5. *Prevention*, October 1980.
6. *Ibid.*
7. *Natural History Magazine*, Spring 1978.
8. *Health Quarterly*, May-June 1982.
9. Natural Food Associates, October 1981.

Index

204

Feinstein, Alvan, 127
Ferguson, Tom, 10, 15, 76
Ferrosilicon concentrate, 24
Fetal development, 117–25
Fever, 10
Fibrocystic breast disease, 14, 44,
  47, 102, 144–47
Fitness in America Study, 57
Flavored coffees, 30
Fletcher, Dean, 121
Fluoride, 68
Folger Coffee Company, 51
Food and Drug Act (1906), 79
Food First Institute, 44
Forney, Robert, 33
Framingham Heart Disease Epide-
  miology Study, 133
Freedom From Arthritis, 152
Freeze-dried coffee, 28–29

Garway, Thomas, 55
Gastrointestinal ailments, 2, 7, 37,
  46, 88, 138, 142–44, 151, 161
General Foods, 28, 49, 51–52
Germann, Donald R., 65–66,
  130–31
Gilliland, Kirby, 12, 138, 141
Glandular exhaustion, 138–39
Goldstein, Avram, 6
Goyan, Jere E., 15–16
Greden, John F., 12, 31
Groisser, Daniel S., 62
Grossman, Morton L., 46
Guarana, 3, 157
G. Washington's Red E Coffee, 28

Haase, Peter, 90
Harris, Mary B., 171
Harris, Seale, 140
*Harvard Medical School Health
  Letter, The,* 140
Headache, 10, 63, 88, 98, 102, 105,
  148–49, 168
Headache remedies, 1, 105, 109
Heart, 2, 7, 10, 12–13, 21, 31, 37–38,
  46, 65–66, 88, 95, 111

Heartbeat irregularities, 133–35
Heartburn, 144
Heart disease, 131–33, 150
Hendler, Nelson, 32
Herbal teas, 14, 57, 69–75, 171–72,
  177
Hershey Foods Corporation, 98,
  101
High Point, 51, 53
Hilker, Doris M., 67
Hills Brothers, 52
How To Get Well, 43, 154
Huggins, Hal, 152
Human Ecology Action League,
  169
Human Performance Laboratory, 9
Hyperactivity, 2, 10, 87–88, 148,
  155

Insomnia, 12, 61, 88
Instant coffee, 22, 27–29, 35, 37, 40,
  65–66, 169
Instant tea, 35, 56, 169
Insulin, 7, 32
Insurance Institute for Highway
  Safety, 33
Internal Flavors and Fragrances
  Bureau, 22
International Coffee Organization,
  15, 27, 36
Iron, 56, 66–68, 90, 97

Jacobson, Michael, 83, 120, 155
Jick, Hershel, 132–33
Josephs, Ray, 24
Journal of Food Science, 44
Journal of Inebriety, 27
*Journal of Norwegian Medical
  Associates,* 48
*Journal of the American Medical
  Association,* 12n, 46
*Journal of the National Cancer
  Institute,* 129

Kaffee H. A. G., 50
Kaizer, Sophia, 6

207

Nestlé company, 28
New England Journal of Medicine, 106, 118, 135, 143
Newsletter of the Institute for Nutritional Research, 4-5
New York Times, 10, 184
Nitrosamines, 79, 111, 130-31
No-Doz, 35, 105-6
NutraSweet, 85*n*
Nutrition Health Review, 24

Only Yesterday, 27
Oral contraceptives, 110, 156
Osteoporosis, 151
Over-the-counter drugs, 1, 16, 105-16, 163-64
Oxalic acid, 56

Paffenberger, R. D., 46, 143
Pain, 60, 88
Pan American Coffee Bureau, 2
Pancreatic cancer, 14, 44, 125-28
Pemberton, "Doc," 79
Pep pills, 1, 105-6, 163
Pepsi, 15, 76, 78, 86
Pepsico, 84
Perrier Company, The, 57
Pert, Candace, 88
Pesticides, 23, 44
Peter, Daniel, 99
Phenylethylalamine, 97
Phenylpropanolamine, 35-36, 108
Philbrick, Diana, 90
Philpott, William, 107, 150
Phosphates, 90
Phosphorus, 153
Physicians' Desk Reference, 154
Phytates, 90
Pierce, Charles, 109
Pocket Guide to Coffees and Teas, The, 38, 61
Popkin, Michael, 109
Postum, 173
Potassium, 22-23, 150
Powers, Hugh, 88

Pregnancy, 90-91, 117-25
Prineas, Ronald, J., 133-34
Procter & Gamble, 28, 51, 53
Prohibition, 27
Prostate, 48, 147
Protein, 56
Pseudoephedrine, 108
Psychodietetics, 141

Quinn, Taylor, 80

Rapoport, Judith, 87, 148
Rapp, Doris J., 88
Redmond, D. E., 8
Red Rose, 62
Regestein, Quentin, 61
Reingold Association, 88
Reproductive disorders, 117-23
Respiratory system, 7-8, 12, 107
Restless legs, 152
Rinzler, Carol Ann, 25, 35
Roberts, Howard, 120-21
Robertson, H. K., 187
Rodale, Robert, 150, 186
Rombout's, 53
Roselius, Ludwig, 50
Royal Crown, 15, 82
Runner's World, 136
Rush, David, 127
Ryan, Kenneth J., 122

Saccharin, 85-86, 91-92
Safeway Supermarket, 52, 84
Salada, 62
San Francisco Consumer Action, 30
Sanka, 22, 49-50, 52-53
S. A. Schonbrunn & Co., 38
Schaal, Stephen, 134
Schauss, Alexander G., 188
Seconal, 122
Sedatives, 110
Segi, Mitsuo, 65
Seizures, 107
7-Up, 15, 78-79, 83, 87, 90

Shedlock, Robert, 52
Sheehan, George, 136
Shorofsky, Morris A., 168
Sickle cell disease, 68
Sleep, 12, 32–33, 56, 61, 88
Slone, Dennis, 132–33
Snyder, Solomon, 8, 46, 138–39
Soda. *See* Soft drinks
Soda Pop, 79
Sodium, 22
Soft drinks, 1–3, 14–16, 47, 76–94,
    134, 155, 157, 163, 180–83
Soil and Health Society, 150,
    186
Sokolov, Raymond, 186
Sperm, 125
Sprite, 87, 90
Stimulant drugs, 106, 113, 163
Stoll, Walt, 88
Stomach, 21, 37, 63, 89, 125
Strictly Female, 35
Strongin, Michael, 146
Sugar, 68, 73, 97, 187
Sullivan, Thomas, 59
Sunkist, 15, 80

Tab, 78, 84–86, 105
Talleyrand, 19
Tannin, 4, 24, 37, 56, 64–68, 71, 90,
    111, 187
Tea, 1, 3–4, 6, 10, 12, 16, 26, 37,
    56–68, 98, 132, 134, 170; caf-
    feine in, 55, 60–62, 69, 71,
    73–75, 157–63; decaffeinated,
    14, 17, 69–73
Tedral, 63
Teeth, 87, 152
Tetley, 62
Thalassemia, 68
Theobromine, 4–5, 8, 55, 61–62, 95,
    98, 101, 125, 139, 145
Theophylline, 4, 8, 55, 61, 63, 95,
    110, 139, 145
Thomas, Robert C., 38
Thompson, Daniel M., 89
Thyroid preparations, 110

Tobe, John, 48
Todhunter, John, 121
Tolerance, 5, 155–56
Toohey, Barbara, 140
*Toxicants Occurring Naturally in
    Foods,* 64
Trager, James, 22, 58, 147
Tranquilizers, 110–11, 141
*Treasury of Natural Health
    Knowledge,* 48
Trichloroethylene, 49–50
Trihalomethane, 86–87, 90
L-tryptophan, 170
Twinings, 62, 159

Ulcers, 89, 98, 111, 143–44, 172
U.S. Department of Agriculture,
    10–11, 16, 57, 86
U.S. Department of Health and
    Human Services, 64
U.S. Food and Drug Administra-
    tion (FDA), 14, 16–17, 23–24,
    35, 44, 49, 51–52, 80–82, 87,
    119–21
U.S. National Academy of Sci-
    ences, 64

van Houten, Casparus, 99
Vegetarian diet, 66, 172
Veterans' Administration, 46
Violent behavior, 98–99
Vitamin A, 97, 151
Vitamin C, 22, 56, 66–67, 72, 111,
    131, 150
Vitamin D, 151
Vitamin E, 151
Vitamins, 37, 56, 60, 150–51,
    170–71, 176
Vivarin, 1, 109

Walden House Drug Rehabilita-
    tion Center, 172
Wall Street Journal, 98
Weathersbee, Paul S., 125
Weight loss, 34–37
Welsh, Philip J., 152

Wetherall, Charles, 32, 69, 144
White Coffee Corporation, 52–53
Wilson's Heritage, 173
Withdrawal symptoms, 8, 148, 155, 168, 170

Yaryura-Tobias, Jose, 98–99
Young, Robert, 42

Zander, Richard H., 137
Zinc, 150, 188